D1553854

TRAVEL WELL
WITH
DEMENTIA

*Essential tips to
enjoy the journey*

Jan Dougherty

Print ISBN: 978-1-54399-310-3

eBook ISBN: 978-1-54399-311-0

A diagnosis of Alzheimer's disease or dementia doesn't mean you have to give up everything you love. For those who enjoy travel, and want to continue to do so, Travel Well with Dementia: Essential Tips to Enjoy the Journey is a must-read both for affected persons and their loved ones. Whether visiting family and friends or venturing to a new location for fun, it's packed with practical tips and strategies that will remove many of the stressors created by travel. This is the first book of its kind that considers what people living with dementia may experience during travel and helps travel companions know what to expect before, during, and after a trip. Find confidence in your ability to stayed engaged with people and places that matter—and continue to create memories!

Embrace the concept that it is possible to live well with dementia, and find joy, purpose, and meaning along the way.

ABOUT THE AUTHOR

Jan Dougherty, MS, RN, FAAN is a nurse leader, innovator, and noted dementia care expert. With over three decades of clinical and leadership experience, Jan has been a pioneer, advancing care for people living with Alzheimer's disease/related dementia and their family caregivers. Many of her program innovations are being used nationally and internationally. She is a noted speaker and author on numerous topics of dementia and has received many state and national awards for her leadership, community service, and program innovations.

An advocate who believes it is possible for people to live well with dementia, she uses her knowledge of dementia and love of travel to educate, guide, and support meaningful travel. With greater awareness and understanding, families, travel companions and the travel industry can join together to ensure successful, safe, and memorable travels for all.

BOOK DEDICATION

To David, my forever companion in life and travel. Your love, support, and encouragement fill my life with the greatest of meaning.

To Katie and Tommy, my two wonderful children who have added so much love and joy to my life adventures.

To the many people living with dementia and family caregivers who have been my teachers, inspiration, and heroes. May you live and travel well through this life.

To Dr. Geri Hall, whose extraordinary knowledge of dementia care and author of the first guide on travel and dementia inspired this book.

And with special thanks to my many dementia care colleagues who have taught, mentored, and guided me in my professional journey.

TABLE OF CONTENTS

Introduction

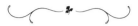

Americans love to travel, spending over $760 billion each year for leisure related travel (www.ustravel.org). For most individuals, travel includes visiting family and friends, while also soaking up the sun at beaches and enjoying shopping and fine dining. Many Americans have a "bucket list" of destinations or experiences hoped to be achieved before traveling is no longer possible. A majority of retirees rate travel as an important aspect in this phase of life. Plus, studies demonstrate that travel is good for our health. A study done by the Transamerica Center for Retirement Studies and the Global Coalition on Aging reported that people who travel are happier than those who don't. Other research suggests travel can also improve mood, lower stress, and enhance relationships.

If that isn't enough, most travelers report getting more exercise (largely walking) on trips than when at home. They also report that travel is mentally stimulating. (To read more about the benefits of travel, download the e-book, "Destination Healthy Travel: the Physical, Cognitive and Social Benefits of Travel" at https://globalcoalitiononaging.com/wp-content/uploads/2018/07/destination-healthy-aging-white-paper_final-web.pdf.)

But what happens when a person begins to have memory and thinking problems and gets a diagnosis of Alzheimer's disease or related dementia? This is a life-changing diagnosis for not only the person but the family, as well. Now affecting an estimated 5.8 million Americans (almost 50 million worldwide), Alzheimer's disease and related dementia is a leading cause of disability (www.alz.org; www.alz.co.uk). Once diagnosed, there's no doubt the idea of travel may seem daunting, if not impossible, for both the person diagnosed and their family.

Yet, travel is not only desired by those affected by these diseases, but it is necessary for many of them. It is important to celebrate milestones such as graduations, weddings, and reunions. An early diagnosis of dementia can also be the genesis of a last-chance dream to take the trip of a lifetime and create lasting memories for the family, as well as an opportunity for the person with dementia to live in the moment.

I have had the privilege of working with people living with dementia, and their families, for over three decades. My work is built on the idea that we can look for strengths and possibilities, rather than giving in to the tendency to focus on deficits and obstacles.

When a new diagnosis is made, the person living with dementia – and their family members – will often reflect on their continued desire to travel. As the disease progresses, family caregivers continue to consult with me about the feasibility of travel, often driven by the desire to allow the person with dementia to join in celebrations. And, on occasion, I have also worked with families who have a deep desire to move their person with advanced dementia back to their home state, to bring peace to their final days and be laid to rest.

In each of these situations, I say, "Yes, we can do this with careful planning!" But there is much to consider. In the business of dementia care, we have an expression: "If you've met one person with dementia, then you have met one person." And so it goes with travel and travel planning. Each person with dementia is different.

Family members will need to craft a unique plan that fits for their person and be realistic and flexible when carrying it out.

This book is not meant to be a review of Alzheimer's disease or related dementias; there are many excellent books and websites providing such detailed information (please see the Resources section at the end of this book). Rather, my goal in writing this book is to provide practical travel tips, tools and guidelines that are much more likely to result in successful travel and happy memories.

I hope that people living with symptoms of dementia and their families can use this guidance to fulfill their desire to stay connected to family and friends, and to find hope, joy and possibilities in each day.

* * *

Since travel means different things to different people, the book uses a "Tips" format to address some of the most common travel needs, from planning to implementation and returning home. You may want to jump ahead and read only the chapters that are relevant to the type of travel you're planning. That approach works just fine.

If you read the book from beginning to end, you are likely to see common and consistent themes throughout. This redundancy is purposeful. My goal is to help you, the reader, to deeply consider these important tips and principles, and to aid you in remembering them.

I have also provided travel stories throughout the book. These stories represent real people and real happenings – both good and bad.

I share them as a way to give concrete examples of how to embrace the positive and keep an open mind even as you anticipate the 'bad' or unexpected things that can and do happen during travel.

You see, I do think that travel is possible for many people living with Alzheimer's and related dementias, but travel advice and planning is absolutely essential to ensure success.

With careful planning and use of the travel tools provided here, I wish you, the reader, every success on your trek!

CHAPTER 1

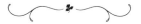

10 Tips for Understanding Dementia Before Travel Begins

Well planned and informed travel always makes for the best trip. Adding dementia into the planning process will change many aspects of travel for both the person with dementia and the family caregiver or travel companion.

In the following chapter, you will find many precautions to consider. This is **not** meant to discourage travel or to create fear. Rather, the goal is to show you that, with careful assessment and comprehensive plans in place, you can ensure the intended travel is successful. Too often, when families and friends have not considered or planned for the added stressors, frustration is the result, and travel is forever ended. While there will come an eventual end to travel for most of us, the goal here is to help you to create a better and more memorable experience.

TIP #1: Dementia is an umbrella term that describes a number of conditions affecting a person's memory and thinking skills and will ultimately impair their ability to live independently

Think of dementia like cancer – it is **not** a specific diagnosis. When we learn that someone has a cancer diagnosis, we ask, "what type?" The question reflects the fact that, for most of us, all we know about cancer is that abnormal cells are growing somewhere in the body. Without a specific diagnosis, appropriate treatment cannot be given, and we can't help the person who has been diagnosed to plan for the future.

The same thing applies to dementia. It is not a specific diagnosis and doesn't lend itself to providing the more detailed information necessary to help the person and their family live their best. There are many different types of dementias, each with differing symptoms and treatments that can also vary according to the type of dementia.

When symptoms of dementia begin to show, it is critically important to get a specific diagnosis such as Alzheimer's disease, vascular dementia, or one of the many other forms of the illness. The specific diagnosis will guide individuals living with dementia – and their family members – to learn more about the condition, including treatment options. It also aids individuals to plan for the future and learn strategies to enhance daily life.

Unfortunately, almost half of people living with symptoms of dementia will never get a diagnosis. Many affected individuals are aware of changes in memory and thinking and are embarrassed by them. However, many of these individuals won't report the changes to a family member or physician for fear of hearing the words "dementia" or "Alzheimer's."

Others living with symptoms will have no insight into their losses. They are not in denial; rather they simply cannot see the difficulties they are having. This is often very frustrating to families who try to point out the changes and get the person to the doctor for a diagnosis.

Caught Off-Guard

Michelle is a devoted daughter who lived at a distance from her parents and made a point to visit each year. She talked to them each week by phone and was aware of her mom's tendency to repeat the same stories again and again. Michelle largely attributed the repetition to her mom getting older – after all, her dad never mentioned anything unusual about her mom.

Unfortunately, Michelle got an unexpected call from the emergency room with news that her dad had suffered a stroke. She caught a flight immediately to join her mom and oversee her dad's care.

Over the coming days, Michelle witnessed firsthand the profound memory loss in her mom. She realized quickly that her mom no longer could cook and needed reminders to take a shower, take her medications and wear fresh clothing. Her mom was unable to remember what had happened to her dad, asking Michelle frequently, "Where is your dad?"

Michelle knew it was time to seek medical advice and assistance. Once her mom was diagnosed with Alzheimer's disease, Michelle and her siblings could use this information to move forward and plan for the assistance required to support both parents.

TIP #2: Alzheimer's disease is the most common type of dementia, but there are many more

Alzheimer's disease accounts for 60-80% of all dementias. Symptoms come on slowly, usually over a period of months to years. People affected begin to first show changes in short-term memory abilities since the memory portion of the brain (the hippocampus) is no longer processing and storing information as in the past. New information is readily lost – but remember, it is not because the person is willfully forgetting. In essence, the brain's 'save' button is broken and new information gets deleted.

Over time, this pattern of forgetfulness begins to interfere with everyday life. Families observe that the person is having more difficulty with common tasks such as managing money and finances, making meals, or attending to household affairs. For those who are still working, work-related tasks take longer to complete, and mistakes happen more often.

Families often voice frustrations that their person is repeatedly asking the same question or telling a familiar story yet again. The affected person will begin misplacing or losing things, often blaming the family for these missing items. Mood can be impacted, as some people become more irritable while others become more passive or withdrawn. The Alzheimer's Association (www.alz. org) provides detailed information about the condition along with many other valuable resources for affected people and family caregivers (please see the Resources section, at the end of this book, for more information).

Vascular dementia is the second most common type of dementia, resulting from small strokes or changes in the small blood vessels in the brain. About 10% of the population will have vascular dementia, often accompanied by a history of high blood pressure, diabetes or another vascular disease.

Symptoms may appear similar to Alzheimer's disease since short-term memory can be affected. However, sometimes the damage occurs in another part of the brain and the person can become confused and disoriented. There may be trouble speaking or understanding language, and some may report vision loss. These symptoms can often also indicate a stroke has occurred.

Stroke-related changes can make the onset of vascular dementia seem more sudden. Yet, over time, changes may have been occurring in the small blood vessels in the brain, causing aspects of impaired thinking to accumulate. Difficulty with planning and problem-solving, sometimes resulting in poor judgment, will begin to appear. You may also witness difficulty paying attention and trouble with word-finding.

Recent brain studies show that vascular dementia often co-occurs with other dementias, including Alzheimer's disease and Lewy Body Dementia. In these cases, the dementia is often referred to as ***mixed dementia.*** For more information, please visit www.alz.org.

Lewy Body Dementia is the third most common type of dementia, with symptoms that look like both Alzheimer's disease and Parkinson's disease. While memory issues appear to be milder than in Alzheimer's, the person will develop features of Parkinson's such as hunched posture, shuffling walk, and more rigid movements.

What is strikingly different about Lewy Body Dementia is the variability in daily function resulting in changes in alertness and confusion. Changes in thinking and reasoning can vacillate from one day to another or even at various times throughout the day. Visual hallucinations, such as seeing people or animals, are very common and are real to the person. Some develop false beliefs (also referred to as delusions) that are simply untrue but seem very true and real to the person. There can be a history of sleep problems, such as REM sleep disorder, that can result in acting out on bad dreams.

These individuals are very sensitive to certain medications. Finally, some will have extreme changes in blood pressure, are prone to constipation, dry eyes, and even sudden falls. For more information, connect with the Lewy Body Dementia Association, www. lbda.org.

Frontotemporal Degeneration (FTD) results from diseases striking either the frontal or temporal lobes of the brain. These disorders are more commonly seen in people between the ages of 40 and 70.

The frontal lobe is often referred to as the "executive center" of the brain. This thinking part of the brain is essential for decision making and appropriate social behavior. When an illness attacks the frontal lobe, the first symptoms usually involve changes in personality, judgment, planning, and social functioning. For example, the person may begin making rude or inappropriate remarks to family or strangers. There are often very poor decisions related to financial or personal matters. They are also more prone to obsessive-compulsive behaviors such as overeating, gambling, or pornography, just to name a few. This frontal lobe presentation is also referred to as "behavioral variant FTD."

For some, the disease will strike the temporal region of the brain. This part of the brain is important for language; thus, problems with language may be among the first symptoms to appear. This can result in the person having difficulty completing sentences or having severe word-finding trouble. For others, it will become impossible to fully understand what is being said. For more detailed information about FTD, visit www.theaftd.org.

TIP #3: Dementias are progressive

Each of the dementias described above is progressive in nature. This means abilities, including memory, thinking, language, function, and mood, will continue to change, typically over a period of months to eight or ten years.

It is often difficult to predict the overall length of the illness, as it varies greatly in affected people. A good rule of thumb is to look back at the differences you've observed over a 12-month period. The rate of change(s) observed during that time will often predict the rate of change you can expect in the coming year.

TIP #4: There are three stages associated with dementia: mild, moderate and advanced

Most dementia experts (physicians, nurses, social workers, and others) often talk about "stages" of dementia. The stages are usually described as ***early-stage Alzheimer's disease*** or ***mild dementia***; ***middle-stage Alzheimer's disease*** or ***moderate dementia***; and ***late-stage Alzheimer's disease*** or ***advanced dementia***.

While the stages of Alzheimer's disease are currently better understood, and are to some degree more predictable, those with vascular dementia and Lewy Body Dementia often experience similar changes over time. Each general stage requires different types of help and assistance, both for the person and for the family caregiver(s).

Table 1

Table 1 provides an outline of expected changes based upon Alzheimer's disease. However, keep in mind that each person is unique and will experience their own changes in a unique way.

As you review the table, place a checkmark next to the feature(s) that seem most consistent with your person. Wherever there are the most checkmarks, that is the likely stage of dementia your person is experiencing.

Table 1: Stages of Dementia		
Mild Changes over 1 – 3 years	**Moderate** Changes over 2 – 5 years	**Advanced** Changes over 1 – 3 years
MEMORY & THINKING		
•Difficulty with short-term memory, concentration and decision making	•Difficulty with short and long-term memory (including visual images) •Growing confusion with simple tasks and remembering relationships and people	•Severely impaired memory for recent and past events, or remembering familiar people
LANGUAGE		
•Problems remembering the right word or name •Decreased reading comprehension	•Increased difficulty expressing self or understanding what is being said • Limited to no reading comprehension	•Unable to carry on a meaningful conversation
MOOD		
•Prone to depression or being socially withdrawn •More self-focused	•Easily upset and frustrated •Prone to making rude or inappropriate remarks	•Appears withdrawn with difficulty interacting/ responding to surroundings or people
FUNCTION		
•Difficulty organizing and managing household affairs, such as cleaning, cooking, and yard work •Trouble handling finances and even making change •Difficulty initiating activities, often appearing disinterested in favorite past activities •Gets lost/mixed-up when driving or walking in familiar places •May be involved in "fender benders" or need someone to navigate when driving	•Needs increased reminders and help over time with the following: **Grooming** - Attention to fine details - Reminders/help for shaving, brushing teeth - Assistance with make-up, hair care **Dressing** - Selecting/coordinating clothing - Sequencing clothing - Buttoning, zipping, snapping clothing **Bathing** - Forgets to bathe and/or denies needing a bath/shower - May become afraid of water in bath/shower **Eating** - Forgets how to use silverware - May lack table manners - Forgets to eat or drink unless prompted - Prefers sweets and soft textured foods **Bladder and Bowel** - Difficulty finding the toilet - Forgets to wipe and/or flush - Prone to incontinent episodes	• Forgets how to walk without help; may lead to eventual loss of body movement •Relies totally on caregivers for: - Grooming - Dressing - Bathing - Feeding - Bladder/bowel •May forget to chew food or swallow

TIP #5: While dementia cannot be cured, it can be successfully managed

Unfortunately, there is no single cure for any of the dementias, and treatments are limited.

- There are four FDA approved medications for the treatment of Alzheimer's disease:

- Donepezil (brand name Aricept)

- Ravistigmine (Exelon)

- Galantamine (Razadyne)

- Memantine (Namenda)

- And a combination of donepezil and memantine (brand name Namzaric).

These medications are often used to treat other forms of dementia. In general, the medications have a modest effect on cognitive symptoms.

There are other symptoms that often occur over the course of dementia that can be managed when brought to the attention of medical professionals. These include depression, anxiety, agitation, sleep, and weight loss. On occasion, some people with dementia will develop psychotic symptoms. These include hallucinations, delusions (fixed, false beliefs), and paranoia. With appropriate medical treatment, these symptoms can also be better managed.

TIP #6: It is possible to live well with dementia

It *is* possible to have a good quality of life while living with dementia. Around the world, dementia friendly communities are developing with the goal of raising awareness and removing stigma to help people to live well with this chronic condition. Learning new ways to manage the day-to-day is essential and will minimize much of the frustration caused by dementia. (These same strategies should be applied during travel and are discussed later in the book.)

For those with a new dementia diagnosis, the Alzheimer's Association and other organizations have created programs to help them (and you) learn how to adapt to the condition. Along with an identified care partner (usually a spouse, adult child, sibling, or friend), it is possible to connect with others and find new, successful ways to live. **This includes travel!** Like other chronic health conditions, learning to accommodate the illness is essential.

TIP #7: The "A" and "D" words can be polarizing – find better words that work for you and the affected person

Much social stigma is associated with the words, "Alzheimer's disease" and "dementia." While each person has the right to get an appropriate and specific diagnosis, there is no need to use these words when talking about the condition, especially if it is upsetting to your person. Some individuals are very forthcoming about their condition, while others find it embarrassing. Because of the added stigma, when family and friends hear these words, they are likely to treat the affected person differently.

Instead, find words that are not upsetting to your person. For example, talking about a "memory loss condition" is often more acceptable. Some will admit to having "trouble thinking." Whatever words your person uses to describe their symptoms, make sure you use them, too.

During travel, you might think about using a Companion Card. An example is shown below. The Companion Card communicates the situation gently, discretely, and effectively – something your person may greatly appreciate.

Sample 1: Companion Card

My family member has a medical condition that affects their memory and thinking abilities.
Your patience is appreciated.

TIP #8: Sharing the diagnosis with family and friends allows for better understanding and support

Hiding the diagnosis from family and friends will not be helpful since those around the person living with dementia will come up with their own (and probably incorrect) conclusions. Unfortunately, without knowledge and understanding, family and friends may stop calling, visiting, or inviting the person to join in usual activities. Social isolation can set in, making things worse for all.

Each person and their care partner must find their own way to share the diagnosis. Keep in mind that some people living with dementia will have no insight into their condition and will deny they have a problem. Others will be very forthcoming and able to tell family and friends how they can be supportive of them over the course of the condition.

As noted previously, when sharing the diagnosis with others, the "A" or "D" words don't need to be used unless you and your person agree to this. Focus on the positive – what the person can still do, enjoys, anticipates, and loves.

Some individuals and their care partners write a letter to close family and friends. Some will hold a family meeting to provide a chance to ask questions, clarify needs, and create a plan to help the person and care partner. Many others may share their condition during a one-to-one encounter with family and friends. You can and should decide which details to share about the diagnosis, based on what others need to know. When planning for travel, it is essential to be transparent about the condition with those who are helping to plan or assist during the trip. We'll address this further throughout the book.

TIP #9: Learning to ask for and accept help is important for both the person and family care partner

Most people living with dementia will experience changing needs over eight to ten years following the diagnosis. This creates growing demands for the care partner who transitions to becoming a full-time caregiver.

In addition to telling close family and friends about the dementia diagnosis, it is essential they learn about the care partner/ caregiver needs as well. While the American culture promotes independence, caring for a person living with dementia requires *interdependence*. That is, we need others to help us along the way. During child-rearing years, most parents find that they need other family members and friends to help them out with rides, babysitting, and variety of other tasks. It's a similar situation when dementia enters our lives: we will all need help.

Learning to *ask for* and *accept* help is a new skill for care partners/caregivers. *It is not a sign of weakness!* I almost never find a family caregiver who says, "I should have waited to ask for help." Rather, most wait too long to honestly tell others what they need and to begin to accept the help that is offered. Start thinking now about how your family and friends can help you. Make a list. Even small tasks such as asking a neighbor to pick up some milk for you can be a godsend.

Likewise, during travel, be honest in your planning about what *you* will need to help your person travel successfully. Whether seeking help from family or friends during travel or from travel professionals (airlines, cruise ships, travel agents, etc.), don't be afraid to ask. You will be surprised how many people will step up to help when you make realistic requests.

TIP #10: Travel is possible with careful planning

For those who love to travel, careful planning often leads to the best and most memorable trips (even when there is no dementia!). When traveling with children, parents usually spend extra hours thinking through the itinerary to ensure the children are well rested, entertained, or distracted so that the entire family can enjoy the trip. While people living with dementia are *not* children, they will benefit from some of the same considerations.

Traveling during the early stage of Alzheimer's disease/dementia will be best. If your person has expressed a desire to take that long-dreamed-of trip, **now** is the time. As the disease progresses to the moderate stage, even greater planning will be needed, and significant modifications made. In the moderate stage, travel **is** still possible; over the coming sections, we will cover in detail how to make those extra accommodations.

Successful travel also requires patience and flexibility. The "best-laid plans" can change rapidly. Challenges can range from the sudden – a delayed or canceled flight, for example – to a person living with dementia who wakes up in a new place and demands to go home. You cannot over-plan travel when considering how dementia may impact your trip.

A Sudden Change of Plans

Maria moved in with her mom, who was diagnosed with early-stage Alzheimer's disease. Her mom grew up in New England and talked with Maria about how she would like to make one last trip home to see her younger brother and a few of her friends. Maria agreed that it was a good idea and made plans for the two of them to fly to Boston, stay in a hotel close to her uncle, and have a daily scheduled visit with a family member or friend.

On the second night of their stay, Maria awoke when she heard her mom in the bathroom. Mom was getting dressed and putting her eyebrows on using a ballpoint pen. Maria was a bit alarmed and asked what her mom was doing. Mom replied, "I don't know what I am doing here. I want to go home."

Maria gently explained that they were in Boston visiting family. Her mom did not accept this and continued to demand to go home. Later that day, Maria and her mom enjoyed a nice visit with her brother, but the next night resulted in the same demand: her mom wanted to go home.

Maria got on the phone with the airline and was able to book a flight home the next day.

CHAPTER 2

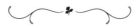

Three Types of Travel Support for People Living with Dementia

There are many travelers who have never before made their own trip plans, simply because they were fortunate enough to have a great travel agent, executive assistant, or competent family member. These valuable assistants clearly have the cognitive abilities to coordinate and execute travel. With Alzheimer's and dementia, you are taking over the role of that competent assistant and handling travel plans yourself.

Table 2

Table 2 outlines the type of travel support you will need to incorporate the many steps involved in independent or assisted travel. There are three distinct types of 'travel ability:'

- **Type #1: Guided travel** calls attention to additional support that will be useful for a person with mild cognitive impairment (or even a frail older adult without memory issues) who will benefit from added time and support.

- **Type #2: Assisted travel** outlines the needs of the person with early-stage Alzheimer's disease or mild dementia when assistance will be needed at various times and touchpoints during travel.

- **Type #3: Dependent travel** outlines the needs of those with middle-stage Alzheimer's disease or moderate dementia, which require a companion at all times.

Use **Table 2** as a guide to begin thinking effectively about the kinds of support you and your person will need to travel successfully and enjoyably. Please note: this table does not address those with late-stage Alzheimer's disease (advanced dementia), since those families will need significant additional medical and physical support.

Table 2. Travel Support for Dementia			
Travel Function	Guided Travel (MCI/General Frailty)	Assisted Travel (Early stage AD/mild dementia)	Dependent Travel (Middle stage AD/ Moderate dementia)
Companion needed?	No. Can travel alone but will generally do better with a companion on a long/ demanding trip	Yes. Will benefit from a companion to assist throughout the trip	Required. Cannot travel without a companion for any part of the trip. May need two companions.
Booking travel/ managing money	-Can make/direct others to coordinate plans & ticketing, seat selection -Can make/direct others to handle payment -May need occasional assistance to calculate a tip, remember to take credit card. etc.	-Needs assistance to make travel plans due to lack of planning skills, including creating travel itinerary and seat selection -Can manage only simple cash/credit card transactions; often needs assistance	- Cannot participate in any travel planning details -Unable to manage money or credit cards
Packing	-Can create/follow a list for packing -Can pack self/direct others to assist	-Needs assistance to create/ follow a list to pack -Will need someone to double-check packing	-Unable to follow a list -Requires someone pack bag(s)
Check-in/ Security	-Generally independent in process -Can request disability services as needed -Manage/direct bags -Can manage own ID/ travel documents (may need a reminder to double check following security)	-Needs assistance for check in process -If flying alone, needs a companion or Sky Cap to escort the person through security to gate/ board and have an escort at the arrival location -Needs flight crew to be aware of assistance that may be required -Needs assistance to direct bags -Will need more time in security with recom- mended wheelchair transport -Will need a companion to assist with travel documents and ID	- Completely dependent on companion for all aspects of check-in -Cannot direct bags -Will need a wheelchair assist to expedite TSA/security -Will require companion to carry all travel documents and ID -Companion must stay with the person at all times and should proceed first in security line so the person does not walk off ahead (in case of not using wheelchair)
Wayfinding	-Able to use navigation tools (e.g. travel monitors) -Can find/seek assistance for gate, toilets, food -Can navigate back to gate, ship, hotel, car etc., with minimum assistance	-Less likely to use monitors or seek assistance to find gate, bus, train, etc. -May become confused when separated from companion with difficulty finding way back to gate, restaurant, car, etc. -Should be watched closely	-Unable to wayfind without companion -Should never be unattended
Boarding/ Transfers	-Independent/obtains pre-boarding assistance -Can find seat -Follows all safety instructions -Exits at designated location and/or uses monitors/seeks assistance for re-boarding	-Needs cueing or assistance in boarding and finding seat -Will benefit from pre-boarding -May not be able to read ticket and follow instructions -Can buckle/unbuckle seatbelt and use the lavatory without assistance -Will require assistance to next plane/gate -If traveling alone, needs reminder to wait for Sky Cap/family assistance	- Requires pre-boarding -Cannot find seat without assistance -Will need help with seatbelt and lavatory -Should not be in emergency exit row -Requires a companion at all times during transfer
Baggage	-Able to identify and collect luggage	-May need assistance to identify luggage	-Requires companion to manage all baggage
Ground transport	-Able to coordinate pick up/hired car service or car rental	-Needs to be met at gate by family or escorted by Sky Cap to family/friends -Unlikely to obtain own ground transport -May walk by a hired driver holding name on poster -Should NOT rent a car for self-driving	-Requires companion to manage all ground transport

CHAPTER 3

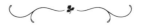

The 10 Most Common Changes in Dementia that Impact Travel

Travel places many demands on the cognitive (thinking) functions of the brain. As symptoms of dementia begin, your person will require more assistance. Depending on which parts of the brain are impacted and the stage of illness, you're likely to encounter a variety of additional challenges. It is imperative, long before you depart, to think through the demands of travel and how the added stress will impact your person.

Families may not fully understand the support that is needed to ensure successful travel – especially when your person doesn't yet have a dementia diagnosis, if they haven't seen the person function on a daily basis, or if they refuse to acknowledge the changes. It is essential to be realistic when you, or a family member, is thinking through the support your person will need.

Change #1: Memory Loss

Memory loss is present in most dementias. In the early stage of Alzheimer's disease (the most common type of dementia), the loss of short-term or recent memory will create challenges in remembering and using new information. During travel, the person may repeatedly ask questions like, "What do we do next?" "What time is the plane leaving?" "Where are we going again?" "What are we doing here?" "When are we going home?"

Although you may have answered the same question just five minutes earlier, your person has already forgotten the answers. Likewise, because of memory loss, your person may be prone to losing things such as travel documents, identification cards, credit cards, etc.

In time, long term memory will also be affected – something that is important to keep in mind when visiting family and friends. Those in the moderate stages of dementia are more prone to forgetting people they have not seen for some time. There can often be confusion about what or who your person is seeing.

Facts and images of events, memories, and people fade, even if the relationships were close. For example, a woman with moderate dementia visiting her older brother may mistake him for their deceased father. She does this because she no longer remembers that her father died and her now-older brother looks just like him.

Memory loss creates many demands on travel and requires that the travel companion be prepared. From planning crucial details to executing daily activities, companions will need to play a very active role. Hang onto important documents, provide reassurance, and answer repeated questions as if you are hearing them for the first time. Don't expect the person with memory loss to keep pace with new information. Accept that your person with memory loss is doing their very best at any time during your trip.

Change #2: Attention and concentration

People living with dementia are much more distractible as the disease progresses, thus their ability to pay attention is diminished. With added noise, new locations, or multiple conversations taking place at the same time, it is imperative to make sure you have your person's attention, especially when providing essential information and instructions. Look directly at your person and give brief instructions so they don't become overwhelmed. Don't rush them – it will only make things more difficult.

Change #3: Slowed thinking

This is very common for affected individuals. They simply require more time to process conversations or written information. It is important to give them time to respond to questions. Watch your person's face for signs of confusion. Restating a question can help, but again – giving them time to answer is still essential.

For example, when going through security lines, ask personnel to only ask one question at a time or give a single command, for example, "Please take off your shoes," or "Please take off your jacket. Put the jacket in the bin for scanning."

Change #4: Lost sense of time

This often happens early in the condition. Repeated questions represent both memory loss and a change in perception of time, also referred to as a 'lost sense of time.' Your person may not realize they just asked this question, told this story or made a similar inquiry just a short time prior.

On long trips, the time to get to the destination may seem eternally long to your person, resulting in repeated questions like, "When will we get there?" Or, a person with early to mild Alzheimer's disease may tell the family, "I am just going to the gift shop and will be back in five minutes," yet might not reappear for a much longer time, causing family members to panic and search.

For those with moderate dementia, the length of the trip can be confusing; you may find your person asking repeatedly, "When are we going home?"

These lost time relationships mean that your person will require additional, gentle time reminders during the day. They will also need a lot more time to get ready each day. ***Rushing your person will create greater frustration and confusion.*** Build extra time into each day and let travel companions or guests know that extra time and patience will be needed during travel.

Change #5: Reading comprehension

This is something that often catches us by surprise. We think the person can read (after all, they can read out loud) but they may not be able to follow through on the next steps due to loss of comprehension. Here's a way to spot a good clue about reading comprehension: notice if unopened mail is piling up or newspapers and magazines go unread. Or, when your person can no longer order off a menu, it's clear that reading comprehension is impaired. It's important because travel requires reading of signs, itineraries, maps, menus and more.

When you notice possible difficulty with reading comprehension, be prepared to support your person. Don't put them in a position where mistakes are likely to be made. For example, don't ask them to find the flight number and gate from a busy arrival/departure screen at the airport. When driving, don't have them navigate using road signs or written directions. If your person is having trouble reading the menu, say, "I see there are a couple of your favorite foods on the menu – a grilled cheese sandwich, and macaroni and cheese. Which one sounds good to you?" Use a dignified approach so your person is not made to feel inadequate.

Change #6: Vision and spatial relationships

Changes in the ability to see and interpret space can change, resulting in many challenges during travel – particularly getting lost. Each year dozens of stories are reported that sound like this: a wife asks her husband to "wait right here" while she uses the bathroom only to find that he is missing when she comes out! When this happens the first time, the wife may think, "He has just gone to the gate or the car," but in fact, he is nowhere to be found.

Memory loss, combined with the inability to pay attention and recognize visual landmarks (like a neighborhood street corner, airport gate or tour bus), or familiar objects (your car), can lead to this kind of confusion. If your person is still driving, they may pass up landmarks they formerly used to navigate – street signs, the corner grocery store and the like – and get lost. Some people with dementia are unable to park in a crowded parking lot because their eye/brain connection doesn't allow them to see the spatial relationships needed to pull the car safely into the parking space. These lost visual relationships can also result in the person driving too close or too far away from the car in front of them.

During travel, be aware of these potential changes so your person doesn't get separated from you or become lost. If your person is still driving, avoid letting them use the car in an unfamiliar location.

Take advantage of public restrooms labeled 'family' or 'disabled,' so you are not separated from your loved one. Bring along an 'Occupied' sign you can hang on the door should you need to accompany your loved one to assist them. Be sure to enroll the person in the MedicAlert/Safe Return program available through the Alzheimer's Association (learn more about it at www.alz.org). If your person has a cell phone, make sure it is fully charged and powered on throughout travel. (You'll find more safety tips later in the book).

Change #7: Planning abilities

Planning and executing everyday activities become much more complex early in dementia, making life a bit more challenging. Successful planning requires the use of short-term memory, time relationships and the ability to focus on details – each of which are changing. There can be difficulty in sequencing steps, even in planning and performing familiar activities. When the person gets confused during a familiar task, asking them to "think about it," can cause even more confusion.

Imagine packing a suitcase for a 10-day cruise to Alaska. In this situation, the person needs to think about a variety of issues including where they are going, for how long, what clothing will be needed, and more. This can be quite overwhelming and during the trip, the family might suddenly realize the person didn't bring along warm clothing, let alone enough underwear!

Be aware that while planning for trips can be very exciting, it can also create a lot of anxiety for people living with dementia. If the person enjoys talking about an upcoming trip and can contribute, then by all means, let them participate. But, if trip planning leads to repetitive questions, growing anxiety, and discussion of not coming along, it is time to end their participation in planning.

Travel companions should try to minimize complex decision-making during travel. Even providing a simple packing list can be helpful to assist the person with memory loss to stay independent. Provide additional time when asking for input; be patient and provide choices whenever possible.

Change #8: Problem solving

Because problem solving draws upon many cognitive skills, it can be an issue in dementia. The greater the detail or complexity involved, the more difficult it will be.

An early change often seen in people with dementia is managing money, since this task is more complex. From balancing checkbooks and reviewing financial accounts to calculating a tip and using cash, there will be growing difficulty and confusion.

In addition, the person will slowly lose the mental agility needed to adjust to changes; likewise, the ability to see a situation for the way it is can also be impaired. For example, a man with mild dementia begins to get lost when driving his car in his local community but believes that he is still able to drive cross-country to visit his son. Not only is his judgment flawed, but he also appears to have no insight into the situation. We can only expect that his ability to problem solve along the way will be impaired, as well.

While some individuals are aware of their difficulty with problem solving, others are completely unaware. Pointing out the situation to those with no insight will only lead to an unwanted argument.

During travel, the person with dementia should not be pressed to problem solve unless provided additional time and a few choices. Don't point out mistakes or errors in judgment; there is no need to cause embarrassment. Simply be a companion to the person and help them feel valued, safe and included.

Change #9: Loss of initiative

Families often report loss of initiative as an early change they see in a loved one. A once very active person may now spend most of the day watching TV and make excuses for not leaving the home. Some will lose interest in favorite activities they've enjoyed in the past. This might also represent depression, which is common in dementia and should be evaluated by a medical provider. However, for many, it simply reflects the changing ability to think of an idea and act upon it. For example, the idea of going to lunch requires the person to formulate a plan: where to go, when to go, who to go with, what to wear, what to order, and how to pay. This can become an overwhelming task, so they made decide it is easier to simply stay home. During travel, the person may say, "I don't feel like going to the museum. You go, I'll just stay here." This is usually met with resistance from the traveling companions who set out to convince or coerce the person into going along.

During travel (and at home), inviting the person to join you in a pleasurable activity or outing will be met with less resistance than asking directly. Instead of saying, "Would you like to go..." (leading to a yes/no response), you might try, "Let's head out now, I have something planned that I know you will enjoy!"

If the person refuses, simply walk away, allow them to forget and then re-approach with another attempt a bit later. Having a Plan B is also essential. There will be times when your person simply is not going to go along with Plan A. Be prepared to adjust your schedule or have a family member, friend, or companion available to keep your person occupied.

Change #10: Inability to consider the needs of others

This is often very difficult for families to see and understand in their loved ones. The 'social filter' can be lost even early-on, leaving the person to speak their mind, talk to strangers, use unwanted language or tell inappropriate stories or jokes. There is a tendency to become focused on their own needs versus those of others. A wife recently told me, "My husband was always such a gentleman, opening doors for me, including my car door. Now he just charges through first!" This is by no means intentional; more than likely, it is just a shift in behavior. He no longer has the same insight into his actions and is now serving his needs before hers.

Since travel is often stressful, your person may be more likely to become impatient in long lines, lectures, or loud environments; the result can be rude remarks. Scolding or correcting your person will not be effective because they see nothing wrong with their behavior. Rather, you, as a companion, should be prepared to manage these situations. Simply hand a simple business size Companion Card (see Sample 1) or note to the impacted party that says, "My family member has a condition that affects memory and thinking. Your patience is appreciated." This is a very effective way to defuse these situations since most people have experienced dementia in a family member of their own.

You can also take these situations as your clue to leave. There is no need to further embarrass your person (or you). Staying longer may only make things worse.

Frequent Flyer

John was a very successful businessman who spent years traveling extensively throughout the world. He was diagnosed with Frontotemporal Dementia at age 57. He had very poor insight into his change in behavior and personality and insisted on continued travel. His wife, Joy, did not know how to curtail his travel and knew he could not travel alone.

Together, they continued to use his first-class travel benefits, but Joy was unable to manage his rude behavior directed at flight attendants and other passengers. She realized that traveling in this manner was no longer an option. It was not a dignified representation of who her husband had been and was embarrassing for her, while also very uncomfortable for the flight crew and other passengers.

As difficult as it was, Joy decided that their days of flying were over.

CHAPTER 4

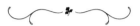

5 Tips for Managing the Added Stressors Created by Travel

As fun as travel is for most, it does create additional demands for all of us. People living with dementia face multiple demands and stressors due to living with an illness that imposes daily challenges in memory and thinking abilities.1 These stressors can be especially difficult when travel companions are not prepared to reduce it or to respond promptly. However, solutions are available to ensure successful travel. Consider the following stressors and solutions:

STRESSOR #1: Fatigue caused by travel

Fatigue is the biggest enemy to the person living with dementia. In a person who already needs more energy to concentrate and remember, fatigue sets in more quickly and adds to confusion. For many, the late afternoon and early evening hours can be the most challenging because of fatigue, a phenomenon known as "sundowning." In addition, fatigue can result in irritable behavior, rude remarks and/or demands to leave or go home.

---

1   Source: Hall & Buckwalter, ***Progressively lowered stress threshold: a conceptual model for care of adults with Alzheimer's disease***, Archives of Psychiatric Nursing, Dec. 1987.

Tips:

- **Be sure the person is well-rested before, during, and after the trip.** During travel, it will be important to create rest periods throughout the day – even when the person insists they are not tired! As a family member or friend, you may need to invite the person to sit quietly with you. In general, experts recommend a 30-minute rest period for every 90 minutes to 2 hours of stimulating activities. While naps are certainly encouraged, a quiet activity such as listening to music, thumbing through a newspaper or magazine, or sipping on a glass of lemonade can be helpful. For the person prone to sundowning, a late afternoon nap can be most helpful in minimizing added confusion.

- **Use the person's best time of the day to enjoy outings and visiting with family and friends.** For most people, the best time of day is usually between the hours of 10:00 a.m. and 2:00 p.m., although you may find your person is less confused even earlier in the day. If possible, try to be are aware of your person's most alert time of day well in advance of travel. Use this 'alertness schedule' as a guide to planning and be sure to communicate these needs accordingly.

- **Be aware of the amount of time your person can enjoy an outing before fatigue sets in.** Trying to cram in too many activities or family visits during travel can become overwhelming. When you see fatigue set in, it is time for a rest period or time to leave altogether. If the person doesn't want to leave, make the departure about you. For example, you can say, "I'm sorry to say I am not feeling well. I think we must go." Be aware that the effects of fatigue can show up sometimes two to three days later and surprise families.

Many caregivers report that coming back from a trip is the most difficult part; it can take upwards of a week to get back to normal. Others report that even when hosting guests at the person's home, when family and friends leave, confusion sets in for several days. Both represent the effects of excess fatigue on the person's brain. Now that you are aware of fatigue – plan for it and be prepared to manage it. (*Please see Chapter 24, 10 Tips for Your Return Home.*)

STRESSOR #2: Ongoing change(s) during travel

Travel – whether you're away from home or welcoming family and friends to visit you – inevitably brings change to the daily routine. With the lost sense of time and changing abilities to plan activities, your person undoubtedly relies on a consistent routine and stable environment to function at their best. Disruption of the daily routine can cause added stress for people living with dementia, along with increased confusion, frustration, anxiety, fear, and even anger.

Tips:

- **It is important to know and honor the person's usual routine and factor it into travel to minimize the inevitable changes.** This is more about keeping activities in the same order each day than by the exact time of day. Waking and bedtime should each be around the same time (adjusting with changes in time zones), eating meals using the routines you've created at home, incorporating rest periods or naps, and planning outings and get-togethers during the person's best time of day.

- **It is essential to communicate with family and friends well in advance about the need to follow the person's preset**

routine. (This is equally important to communicate to guests who are traveling to visit you.) Educate your travel companions about the need for routine or they may interpret routine as unnecessary rigidity, and will not be prepared to adjust their schedules, as well. This added resistance will add to your stress, too!

Staying on Schedule

Bill and Marilyn have always enjoyed travel, both domestically and internationally. Marilyn had learned the importance of building a routine for Bill since his diagnosis of vascular dementia. They decided to join a small group of friends to tour the South; the prospect of added support made this trip seem possible.

One of the couple's daily routines included attending morning Mass at their Catholic parish followed by breakfast at home. Because of the time change on this trip, Marilyn and Bill went to breakfast in a new location before heading off to church. However, following Mass, Bill became very insistent on having breakfast, which was going to interfere with the plans for the day. Marilyn tried, without success, to convince Bill that they already had eaten but quickly realized Bill would need to have a second breakfast to support his usual routine. They would simply join up with their friends later that day.

Fortunately, their friends were very understanding and adjusted the rest of their trip to allow for a later Mass followed by breakfast each day.

STRESSOR #3: Misinterpretation of the environment and feeling overwhelmed

People with memory and thinking problems lose the ability to properly interpret what they see and hear, particularly as the disease progresses and when fatigue is present. Noises and images can become distorted and misinterpreted. These changes lead the person to become uncomfortable in crowds or noisy settings. A large group or excess noise, especially when coupled with fatigue, can result in an angry outburst, a demand to leave, or rude statements. Even at family gatherings, when a child is loud and rambunctious, the person with dementia may yell, "That child is a brat!"

When staying at a different location than home, people with moderate dementia are more prone to misinterpret their current environments, particularly in the evening. Shadows and even pictures on the wall may be interpreted as others being present in the room. New sounds, to them, might mean someone is breaking into the room. This is a time for patience and watchful companionship, knowing your person is confused and anxious.

Tips:

- **It is important to recognize when the person is overwhelmed.** This may include observing the person withdraw from the activity or communication altogether, appear to be more confused, make rude remarks or demand to leave. When this happens, it is time to either get to a quieter location or leave. Encouraging the person to stay at the gathering may result in unwanted behaviors or waking up with added confusion during the night or the next day.

- **When confused by the environment, provide reassurance by letting them know they are safe, and that you will stay with them.** Let your person know you have things under control by using language like, "I have called security and they are taking care of the situation." It doesn't help to argue with the person or try to orient them to this new reality. Acknowledge the upset and provide a pleasant distraction such as eating a favorite snack, turning on a favorite TV show, listening to familiar music, talking about a nice memory, etc. This may also be an indication that the trip may be over and it is time to return to the comfort and routine of home.

STRESSOR #4: Too much demand on the person

Too much of any one thing during travel can add unwanted stress since your person will try to keep pace. For example, a long, hard-to-understand lecture in a museum may lead to rude comments or wandering off. Some individuals may think they can participate in activities that have become restricted at home, such as driving. On a demanding tour, a person may announce that "I am not coming along" when the bus is leaving and all must be boarded!

Sometimes the family believes the person can do something that they can no longer do. For example, perhaps your person cannot order from a menu since they can no longer remember or understand what each item is, let alone recall if they like that particular food. Or, the person is given too many choices and can't decide due to confusion.

Tips:

- **Accept that the person is trying to do their very best.**

- **Try to go with the flow, providing a pleasant distraction and avoiding arguments.**

- **Avoid providing lengthy explanations or reasoning with the person**. This will add to the overwhelm.

- **Implement Plan B** (in other words, what else can you do *right now* to ease the frustration?)

- **When planning travel, factor in how demanding the itinerary will be on your person**. If it is too much and the itinerary cannot be flexible, this may not be the trip for you.

- **Ask about the length of outings, lectures, tours, etc.** Those with early-stage Alzheimer's disease/mild dementia can tolerate up to two or three hours of a stimulating activity, while those with moderate disease may only be able to tolerate up to one hour. Be aware of how much your person can handle before putting them in a situation that creates too much demand on their abilities.

STRESSOR #5: Health issues

Many people living with dementia have other chronic health conditions that must also be kept in mind during travel. Should the person become ill during travel, the companion will see the person develop sudden and worsening confusion, disorientation, and even hallucinations. Even a medication like scopolamine, used to prevent seasickness, can cause sudden confusion. Sudden and increased confusion is often referred to as "delirium" and should be considered a medical emergency. Should this occur, families should not delay and should seek local medical treatment immediately.

Tips:

- **Seek immediate medical attention if you see sudden/worsening confusion.**

- **Carry a complete list of over-the-counter and prescribed medications and dosages, along with pharmacy number(s).** In addition, the family should have the person's medical providers' names and phone numbers. (Please see Table 3: Sample Medication List.)

- **Let the treating medical provider know about the person's dementia diagnosis.**

- **Always carry your person's insurance card(s) with you during travel.** If you are on a Medicare Advantage plan, you may want to inquire about health care coverage out of the area, since there may be limitations.

- **Consider purchasing travel medical insurance when traveling domestically or abroad.**

CHAPTER 5

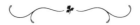

10 Reasons to Reconsider
or Avoid Travel

There are times when people living with dementia should NOT travel. Families must carefully consider and reconsider travel, particularly when the best options may require medical expertise and/or medical transport. There are also times when the family may not be in a position to manage travel for the affected person. Here are 10 reasons to question whether this is the right time to travel:

REASON #1: Severe confusion

As discussed previously, as dementia progresses, confusion will worsen. Travel will be challenging if not impossible when:

- Your person is unable to recall or recognize the family member or travel companion.

- Your person cannot follow instructions and/or becomes agitated or upset when pressed.

- Your person has persistent disorientation, confusion, and is easily upset, even in familiar places.

- At home, your person repeatedly asks to go home and no longer recognizes their own home.

REASON #2: Psychosis is present and upsetting to the person

Progressive dementias can cause the brain to play tricks on the person, especially for those with a diagnosis of Lewy Body Dementia. When this happens, the person may see things that are not there (hallucinations), believe things that are not true (delusions), or believe that someone is out to harm them (paranoia). Hallucinations, delusions, and paranoia are all considered to be symptoms of psychosis.

For some, these symptoms can be quite mild and not terribly disruptive while others may find them very upsetting. When they come on suddenly, *it often indicates that a medical condition is out of control*. The person will need help immediately and should be seen by a medical professional.

Travel should be reconsidered when the following is present or observed on a routine basis:

- Your person is seeing things (usually people or animals) that are upsetting to them and they cannot stop thinking or talking about it.

- Your person is fixated on something that is not true and is very upset by it.

- Your person believes that someone is trying to cause harm or steal from them.

REASON #3: Mood issues

Dementia affects a person's ability to manage their emotions. For some, the type of dementia (for example, Frontotemporal Degeneration or FTD) limits their ability to cooperate or to mind their manners or words. The inability to plan ahead and manage time relationships can be very upsetting for some. And, when the caregiver is absent, the person may become quite anxious.

Additional considerations that might exclude travel include:

- Your person has extreme anxiety or restlessness resulting in the inability to sit for extended periods.

- Your person gets upset easily in crowded, noisy settings.

- Your person yells, screams, swears, or cries spontaneously.

- Your person has consistent rude and/or inappropriate social behavior.

REASON #4: Physical concerns

Since the majority of people living with dementia are older, they may have physical limitations that make travel more challenging. Reconsider travel for your person when:

- They are at risk for or have had frequent falls. If you decide to travel, you will need to order a wheelchair to use during your trip to avoid injury.

- They have incontinence that cannot be managed over pro-longed travel. While incontinence products have improved greatly, family restrooms are not the norm and sitting in a wet brief is uncomfortable (and worse yet, smelly – remember, as a companion, part of your responsibility is to help preserve their dignity). (Please see Chapter 11, *10 Tips for Managing Continence During Travel.*)

- They are prone to physical or verbal outbursts that include hitting, spitting, yelling or swearing. Unfortunately, we live in a world of growing intolerance for certain kinds of behaviors that can be misinterpreted as a threat to others.

REASON #5: Medical condition

It is estimated that about 90% of people living with dementia will have at least one or more additional health conditions.2 While most stable and well controlled chronic health issues like diabetes and arthritis can be managed, there are other health conditions that can make travel more challenging. It is essential to seek advice from the treating medical professional before taking a trip. Travel is not advised when any of the following health conditions are present:

- Congestive heart failure

- Unstable angina (chest pain)

- Recent heart attack

- Recent surgery

- Recent deep vein thrombosis or pulmonary embolus

- Any *unstable* medical condition

REASON #6: Family caregiver/travel companion is unable to handle the person's changing behavior

Caring for a person with dementia can be tough. The 24/7 demands can leave the caregiver fatigued and stressed – especially when that person is alone in providing care. Without a team of family and friends to help, the family caregiver is more prone to their own upset.

Adult children and other family and friends who are not in touch with the caregiver on a regular basis may be completely unaware

---

2　Co-morbidities in dementia: time to focus more on assessing and managing co-morbidities, Age & Ageing, Volume 48, Issue 3, May 2019, https://academic.oup.com/ageing/article/48/3/314/5421357

of the caregiver's health and well-being. They may not take into consideration that the caregiver is not well-equipped to handle the situations that can arise during travel.

What's worse is that Alzheimer's disease and related dementias continue to be underdiagnosed worldwide. ***It has been reported that nearly half of Medicare beneficiaries with a dementia diagnosis will never be told about the diagnosis by their medical provider***.3 Caregivers may also be kept in the dark. As a result, the family caregiver may perceive that the affected person is just being difficult, belligerent or childlike.

When selecting a travel companion to accompany the person living with dementia – whether the companion is paid or is another family member – it is important to assess their ability to calmly respond to difficult situations that may occur.

The following situations or responses by the family caregiver or identified travel companion can indicate they may not be well suited for a trip that includes your person:

- The caregiver becomes easily upset or embarrassed when their person says/does something humiliating.

- The caregiver scolds or corrects the person in front of others.

- The caregiver tries to argue or reason with the person over situations that don't matter.

- The caregiver uses excess alcohol (or other substances) to deal with the stress of caregiving.

---

3   2019 Alzheimer's Disease Facts and Figures, Alzheimer's Association, https://www.alz.org/media/documents/alzheimers-facts-and-figures-2019-r.pdf

The caregiver openly expresses anxiety about traveling with the person.

Frustration for All

Jane and Bill are retired university professors who have always enjoyed educational tour groups. Jane was excited when she was presented with an opportunity for the two of them to join a group of like-minded travelers on a 10-day trip to Cuba.

Early into the trip, it became quite evident to others that Bill was very confused. He asked repeated questions, had difficulty following instructions and at one point became separated from the group when he went off on his own to use the bathroom.

As the trip progressed, Jane became increasingly frustrated with her husband. She began scolding him in front of the entire group when he would wander off or repeatedly ask the same question of the guide. Bill was initially embarrassed when being corrected by Jane. However, in time, he began yelling at her when she attempted to correct or reason with him.

Fortunately, another person on the trip who had cared for a parent with dementia was able to take Jane aside and provide tips to help her be more patient with Bill. This kind traveler also respectfully talked with others in the group about how they could each befriend Bill and help him feel more successful on the trip.

**This story represents that many times dementia goes undiagnosed as the person has no insight into their loss(es) and/or the family may minimize the memory and thinking changes or think they are normal age-related changes. In this case, Bill visibly had changes consistent with dementia.

REASON #7: Family caregiver is unable to accept the person's limitations

Many family caregivers are never educated about their person's dementia diagnosis. Without understanding how this progressive condition will affect their loved one, they will likely have unrealistic expectations about their person's ability to travel.

Often, it is extended family and friends who "don't get it." They only speak to the person living with dementia via phone and think what they're hearing are normal symptoms of aging. They may not believe what the family caregiver is sharing about their loved one's changing abilities or think the caregiver is making too much of it. Some spousal caregivers may hide this information from their adult children because they don't want to be a bother.

It is not uncommon, when family members come to visit the person with dementia, that the individual rises to the occasion and seems fairly normal. However, the truth is the adult children are not there to witness the meltdown that happens after they leave (Please see Chapter 23, *10 Tips for Your Return Home*).

There is often a lot of pressure for the person living with dementia and their caregiver to attend celebrations that involve travel, such as graduations, weddings, and holiday gatherings. Families may dismiss the caregiver's concerns and warnings that travel is difficult for their loved one. Or, there may be resistance when the caregiver asks that the family celebration be modified so that their person may participate.

One of the most common issues reported during travel is when the person living with dementia goes off on their own to use the bathroom, then becomes confused and gets lost. Likewise, the caregiver may ask their person to wait while they use the restroom. Because the person quickly forgets why they are waiting, they walk away to look for their family member and become lost.

Missed the Boat

Al and his companion, Marsha, had been talking for over a year about taking a European river cruise. After Al had been diagnosed with mild Alzheimer's disease, the couple decided it was time to make the trip. Marsha had a very poor understanding of his condition and was not prepared for what would happen. The couple seemed to be enjoying their trip when one afternoon Marsha decided to take a nap and Al announced that he would go out and "explore."

Al was not only unable to track time and return to the ship before departure but lost his way when he was out and about. The cruise departed and an hour later Marsha awoke but thought Al was enjoying a cocktail in the lounge.

After dark, she became concerned when Al did not return to the room. She frantically searched the ship – but no Al. Finally calling security, the search for Al began. After 36 hours, Al was located by the local police in the outskirts of Amsterdam. He was cold, dehydrated and thoroughly confused. Marsha took a plane to meet him and, after being discharged from a hospital, the two made their way back to the U.S.

REASON #8: Family caregiver's own health issues

When we look at the impact of caregiving on the physical and emotional health of those providing important care to others, the statistics are staggering. According to the Family Caregiver Alliance (https://www.caregiver.org/), the demands of caregiving can cause the caregiver to neglect their own wellness, putting them at greater risk for serious health issues like heart disease, cancer, diabetes and depression in particular. ***Sadly, spousal caregivers are 63% more likely to die while caring for a person with dementia.***

Before considering travel, you, as the caregiver, should be boldly honest with yourself to determine if you are up for the trip. This is especially true if you must keep vigil should your person try to leave the room unattended at night or need constant companionship. Extended family and friends should also consider this demand on you, the primary family caregiver, before asking you to travel.

REASON #9: Family caregiver/travel companion is unprepared

Sometimes, even when there is a known dementia diagnosis, the family does not carefully consider how the person will do during travel. This is especially true if the person living with dementia is pleasant and cooperative most of the time. The caregiver might assume that the person will still be able to go with the flow despite the radical change in location(s) and routine(s) caused by travel.

Most family caregivers become very independent as they go about their duties and do not want to impose on others to help them out. So, the idea of asking a paid or unpaid companion to assist with travel seems silly to them. Even when another family member offers to assist in making a trip, this may be met with resistance from the caregiver.

In any of these circumstances, it is essential to evaluate the family caregiver's ability to safely travel and be a companion the person with dementia.

Sharing the Care

Debbie and her sister, Sue, agreed to share the care of their mom, Betty, who was living with progressing Alzheimer's disease. Because they lived in different states, they arranged for Mom to fly alone on a non-stop flight from Baltimore to Phoenix.

Due to some unexpected issues that occurred during flight, the plane was re-routed to Albuquerque. The flight crew was uninformed of Betty's diagnosis and her need for support and supervision. After landing, an airline employee found Betty wandering in the airport.

Luckily, the airline staffer was able to eventually make contact with the daughters. New arrangements were made, and Betty finally arrived safely in Phoenix. However, the added stress for Betty and her daughters (not to mention airline personnel) underscored the fact that Betty could not travel alone.

REASON #10: The person's or caregiver's medical provider refuses to give medical clearance to travel

Although travel is not always possible, there are solutions. Families and friends can come to visit the person with memory loss and their caregiver. Perhaps they might even offer to stay with the person and give the caregiver a break.

By using music, food, and stories, family and friends can create a sense of travel, using the imagination to transport the person living with dementia to a special place and create moments of joy. While the person will quickly forget the event in the days and weeks to come, family and friends will remember them for a lifetime.

Likewise, the family caregiver may enjoy a much-needed leisure trip or the opportunity to join in an important celebration. In these situations, 24-hour companion care at home from a family, friend or paid companion might be an option. Or, arranging for a respite stay in a residential care setting can make travel possible for the family. (*Please see Chapter 15, 10 Tips for Finding Respite Care Options.*)

Recreating the Travel Experience

Cathy developed early-onset Alzheimer's disease in her mid-fifties. With a college background in art history and French, she and her husband Don had always dreamed of going to Paris. However, rearing five children and meeting the demands of daily life prevented this dream from coming true.

Cathy would occasionally mention to her family her desire to visit Paris, but as the months became years of living with dementia, it appeared this dream would no longer be a reality for Cathy. That is until her family decided to bring Paris to her!

Cathy's family got together and planned an elaborate celebration, creating a night in Paris right in their backyard. Lights were strung about the yard with backdrops created of popular Parisian landmarks. An accordion player created the ambiance with music and a French-inspired meal was served to all. Cathy was safe and sound, experiencing Paris and surrounded by a loving family who witnessed her living joyfully in the moment. They, too, savored this celebration of life and love without the added stress of travel.

CHAPTER 6

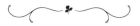

10 Tips for Successful Travel Planning

The best trips are those that are well thought out and **planned in advance**. You've learned that, with accommodations for the person living with dementia, travel is feasible. You also understand that sometimes travel may not be in the person's best interest (or yours!).

By using the following travel planning tips, you will be prepared to take your trip or to host family and friends who come your way for a visit.

TIP #1: Determine the purpose of the trip

Purposeful travel makes for the best travel. If this is a bucket list trip for you or your person, determine if it truly makes sense. If the purpose of the trip is to visit family for pleasure or an upcoming event, carefully evaluate what is needed and set clear expectations. Honestly ask yourself, "*Is my person a willing and able participant?*"

As mentioned previously, early in dementia, travel is much more doable. Your person is probably much more likely to participate in a bit of planning and enjoy the trip itself. But as dementia progresses, and the person is no longer talking about taking a much-desired trip or does not remember the grandchild who is about to be married, it may not make sense to plan the trip, let alone take it. In this instance, you may want a family member to stay with your loved one or consider using a respite option (please see Chapter 15, 10 Tips for Finding Respite Care Options).

TIP #2: Consider the travel demands

Now that you've outlined the purpose of the trip, you should next ask yourself, "Can the demands of the trip be modified in a way to ensure it is successful?" This includes asking:

- **How long can you or your person truly tolerate being away from your home**, the most comfortable place of all? As your person's condition progresses, shorter trips will be more successful. The longer a trip goes on, the more likely your person is to become confused.

- **Where will you be visiting and staying?** Keeping a 'home base' will help your person be more comfortable. Cruise vacations can be a great choice because they provide a consistent room. Likewise, when visiting family or friends, staying in the same location for the entire trip (whether it is a hotel or in a family member's home) will be best. If your nightly stay changes frequently, you may want to re-think the trip.

- **In general, the quickest mode of transportation to arrive at your destination is the best.** For a road trip, ask yourself, "Can my person tolerate a multiple-day destination by car?" (Please see the detailed tips on air, road, and cruise travel contained in Chapters 19, 20 and 21.)

TIP #3: Determine if your person can handle the travel demands

By now, you have realized that you must be in charge of most, if not all, the details. Travel is exhausting for all of us, so are you really up for the task? If not, time to re-think the necessity of the trip. Or, consider hiring a travel companion or asking a family member to accompany you.

As you begin to appreciate how the demands of travel will impact your person, how confident do you feel in your ability to problem-solve as challenges arise? Are you comfortable asking for help? Are you willing to sit out an excursion or family event on a bad day? Putting your needs first is not selfish. Without your ability to anticipate and be flexible in making needed changes during travel, the trip will not be successful. Be fair to yourself in thinking through what you need.

TIP #4: Consider whether or not to include your person in planning

This is a tough one. It seems inconsiderate not to include your person in planning, especially if he or she enjoyed planning trips in the past. Please understand that excluding your person from the planning is by no means a sign of disrespect. Rather, you are acknowledging that planning has become more difficult and can create unwanted stress for your person. This may mean that, at times, you may not want to ask the person if they want to come along – especially if you know the answer will be "No!" However, that kind of feedback can be useful in the overall decision whether to go or not.

Early on, many people living with dementia will enjoy participating in the planning. Having booklets to look at can help in the planning process since it provides some structure for your person. Later, as you observe more confusion and/or anxiety around time relationships, you may want to re-think if and when to include the person in planning.

For example, you might announce to your loved one that you are going to a grandson's graduation that is several months away. Suddenly, you find your person constantly asking when you are taking this trip. This is probably time to decrease the stress for both of you and stop involving them in these kinds of decisions.

TIP #5: Create reasonable expectations

As a care partner or family caregiver, you understand the demands of daily life. For example, a family reunion at sea may sound great to some family members; yet, as the caregiver, you know your person does not do well outside of her usual routine and environment. It's important to communicate this change openly and honestly with family members.

Or, let's say your person is able and willing to join along in the reunion at sea. Will family members be receptive when you opt out of a planned excursion or dinner because your person is having a bad day? Are there other family members who are willing to assist you and your person, so you can have some time to yourself or with other family members without your person present?

These same principles apply when family and friends come to visit you. Ask yourself these questions:

- Can my person tolerate the added stress of visitors staying with us?

- Do the visitors understand what my person's routine is like and how they can support it?

- Do they know how to include my person in conversations, dining out, and other events?

- Have I openly and honestly explained what I need for the visit to be successful?

Help others know what to expect and tell them how they can help and support you and your person.

> **Communicating Expectations**
>
> Sam and Marilyn have always loved to have their kids come and visit them. However, Sam noted that after the last visit from their daughter and her family, Marilyn had some very bad days. Since he now was assuming the daily tasks of cooking and laundry – something Marilyn had previously always enjoyed – he was aware her Alzheimer's disease was progressing.
>
> Sam recently got a call from one of the kids who was excited to share plans for an upcoming trip to visit the couple. However, as much as Sam was looking forward to a visit, he was struggling with how to share with them that he and Marilyn could not host the family in their home, nor could they expect Marilyn to cook the favorite meals as she had in the past.
>
> Sam consulted with a social worker at the memory clinic who encouraged Sam to write a letter to all the children. In the letter, he explained Marilyn's condition and the additional care she required. He honestly communicated his desire to stay connected to the children and grandchildren and told them how much he appreciated visits.
>
> He laid out his needs for their future visits: getting a hotel room; planning visits with the couple during Marilyn's best time of the day; staying in for meals, and; providing help with cooking meals. Sam asked his children to call their mom frequently just to say "hello" and tell her how much they loved her. He asked for their understanding and support of these changes.

TIP #6: Consider ease and upgrades

If you have never considered yourself to be a first-class passenger, now is the time to start. You want to minimize your stress, so you do not unintentionally add to the stress of your person.

Consulting with a travel agent can be helpful – they are skilled at thinking through paid 'add-ons' that perhaps you have never taken advantage of or considered (*please see Chapter 16, 10 Tips to Using a Travel Agent*).

For example, pay-ahead options may make for a quicker check-in to your hotel or pick up of a rental car. Flying business class or paying for a premium economy seat will give you extra time, comfort, and legroom on planes that are consistently filled with too many passengers. Perhaps you want to send your luggage to your destination ahead of time to minimize your wait in the airport. Or maybe a car service is best to whisk you directly to your hotel, so you can get the rest that you and your person need.

Think of your time and your person's travel abilities as a premium. Treat yourself like you are an executive who must optimize every opportunity to make the travel successful.

TIP #7: Factor in flexibility

A trip rarely goes as planned – even without dementia. Travel author Rick Steves has a "no grumpiness allowed" policy for those who take his trips. This should apply to all who travel.

Expect that there may be things you planned that do not work out. Instead of getting frustrated (or "grumpy"), be ready to shift your plans. Your ability to be flexible, go with the flow and accept things that go wrong will be critical to your success. And since your person is carefully watching you and your body language, when they see that you are staying calm, they will stay calm as well. Conversely, if you start getting worked up, so will they – but they may not understand why.

TIP #8: Create a backup plan

Planning ahead is key to staying flexible. Be sure to craft backup plans (Plan B, C or even D) in case the trip does not go as you had hoped.

For example, will the land tour you booked allow you and your person to opt-out and stay at the hotel for the day, should added rest be necessary? If the wedding you are attending is in the evening, will your family understand that you will not be joining the family luncheon? If you need to leave your trip early, do you know how you will arrange a sudden change in travel plans?

Don't be caught off guard. It's better to have a backup plan ahead of time so you are ready to jump into action.

TIP #9: Consider a staycation

Perhaps it has been a while since you traveled, and you are not sure how your person will handle it. A staycation (i.e. a mock vacation in your own town) may be a great way to test out how adaptable you and your person might be should you want to take a longer trip.

Find a hotel in your area – ideally one with additional amenities such as a pool and lounge area, a restaurant on the property, or a refrigerator in the room for beverages and snacks. Book a room for two to three nights and then treat yourself to the local area, much like you would if you were a visitor. During your stay, try to keep your usual routine. If your person seems to enjoy this brief trip away from home, it may indicate that a longer trip may be success-ful. Likewise, if they wake up at night and are confused and afraid, it may tell you that traveling is not in their (or your) best interest.

TIP #10: Get extra help and/or accommodations lined up in advance

As you plan your upcoming travel, be realistic about needing help during the trip. It is better to have extra help and not need it than to be caught in a situation that requires more than you can handle.

For example, ask a family member to join you to help you with your loved one. Be clear about how they can assist you during the trip.

When this is not feasible, consider hiring a companion or aide, especially if your person needs assistance for grooming, dressing or bathing. In these situations, you will want to share, ahead of time, what your person needs and how the aide can best assist you. Do not think the aide will just figure it out. What may seem obvious to you will not be obvious to others. (Please see 10 tips to Hiring a Travel Companion.)

If you are unsure whether your person will be comfortable staying at a family or friend's home, you may want to book a room in a local hotel as a backup plan. Let friends or family know in advance you are doing this and why it is needed. This will avoid confrontation and hurt feelings should you need to activate this 'Plan B.'

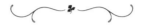

CHAPTER 7

10 Tips for Visiting Family and Friends (at Their Place or Yours)

Visiting family and friends ranks as one of the main reasons people travel. Maintaining these connections is important for people living with dementia and for those they love. As we have mentioned throughout the book, it is important to plan for these get-togethers and make sure that expectations for the visit are understood by all. When family and friends have the information they need, they are more likely to be helpful and to ensure that the visit goes well.

A Great Reunion

Julie and Mick were high school sweethearts who maintained a strong friendship with Mick's best friend, Joe. When their 50th high school reunion approached, Joe was quick to ask Julie if she and Mick would consider coming back home for this gathering. Julie expressed some reservations; although he had always been a friendly and fairly easy-going guy, Mick was now living with dementia and had growing confusion. Joe was aware of Mick's condition and told Julie he would be sure to stay close to Mick during the entire weekend so Julie could relax and enjoy visiting with some of her old classmates.

During this four-day trip, Joe was true to his word. He and Mick enjoyed visiting some of their old hangout spots during the day and Joe made sure Mick got some needed rest every afternoon. On the night of the class reunion, Joe accompanied Mick as they made their rounds to see old friends. The name tags worn by each of the former graduates helped Mick tap into his remaining social skills and interact with all. In fact, most people did not even recognize Mick's dementia.

The three of them returned to their hotel laughing and discussing what a fun night it had been. Mick turned to Julie and Joe and asked, "Who the hell were all these people?" They all shared a laugh because even Julie and Joe had forgotten some of their peers.

Julie held this reunion close in her heart, still seeing the same old Mick she knew and loved. And she was forever grateful for the assistance of their dear friend Joe.

TIP #1: Get details from family and friends before the trip

Whether you and your person are traveling to visit family or friends, or they are planning to come and see you, the first thing to determine is the length and purpose of the trip. Perhaps you live in a sunbelt state and your grandkids want to come out for spring break and take in a few ballgames. Maybe you are traveling to see your granddaughter get married. You will probably want to know about any additional festivities that are planned during either visit. ***Don't be afraid to probe for more details.*** This will allow you to be more prepared when making arrangements either at home or away.

TIP #2: Determine if the visitors should stay with you or get a hotel room

Too much commotion and noise can quickly overwhelm the person living with dementia. This might include too many people in one place; a guest who talks non-stop; a TV blaring in the background; grandchildren making a lot of noise as they play; or family members who expect you to join in all the festivities. Each of these situations may be too much for your person to handle.

Keeping your person's routine intact is most helpful during visits, along with some planned quiet or rest periods. Yet, this can be difficult, too, whether you're staying with family or friends or vice versa.

If you determine that your person will become overwhelmed, communicate in advance with family and friends. Help them to understand why they cannot stay with you or why you are getting a hotel room.

If they insist on staying with you, be clear with them about what they must do. For example, let them know your person's routine, and ask them to create a reason to leave during a predetermined rest period. Let them know you will need their help to make meals, do dishes, laundry or meet any other demands you think may arise.

If your person asks you why family or friends are not staying with you, simply say, "This is a vacation for them, as well. They wanted to enjoy some free time."

TIP #3: Communicate in advance about your person's needs

Letting family and friends know in advance about your person's condition is an important factor in making the trip successful and setting realistic expectations. Some family caregivers will send periodic updates to family and friends to keep them informed. They may send copies of handouts from educational programs or even links to helpful websites. Others have sent medical provider notes so that the entire family has the same information about the person living with dementia. ***Unless family members or friends understand how dementia is impacting your person, they will not understand and will not be prepared.***

TIP #4: Help family and friends support the person's daily routine

If you have read this book from the start, you know by now that structure and routine help your person live their best. You've also learned that those who are not caring for someone living with dementia probably do not understand or appreciate how important planning, structure, and routine can be.

It is always best to inform family and friends in advance of the routine that works best for your person. If they want to regularly include you and your loved one in activities, ask them to think about how they can adapt their schedules to accommodate your person's routine.

Let them know things like:

- What time you and your person are ready to start your day

- When you eat your meals

- Any usual rest periods

- Nighttime rituals

- Favorite activities (TV shows, card games, etc.)

TIP #5: Try to schedule gatherings and outings during the person's best time of day

Most people living with dementia do best between the hours of 10:00 a.m. to 4:00 p.m. But each person is different. For some, there is more confusion in the morning and the day gets better as it goes. For many, evening hours are more difficult because of growing fatigue (this goes for most of us!). As you have helped your family and friends know about your person's condition, you can help them be flexible in scheduling events and gatherings.

While in the past you may have celebrated Thanksgiving dinner at 4:00 p.m., you now understand that this is not a good time of day for your person. Instead, you ask your daughter or son if dinner could be moved up to 1:00 p.m. so that you can plan to leave by 4:00 p.m.

Maybe your friends love to go out to lunch but you know that a loud and crowded restaurant is very upsetting to your mom and she is going to demand to leave. Let them know you would prefer to join them for lunch at 11:00 a.m. or after 1:30 p.m. to miss the crowds.

On a cruise, you know that joining your family for a 9:00 a.m. large group excursion is way too early. See if they might consider booking an 11:00 a.m. private family tour instead.

Aimed with this knowledge, your family and friends are more likely to adapt their plans so you can join in the fun.

TIP #6: Let family and friends know how they can help you and your person during the visit

Sometimes we are too quick to share what the person can no longer do versus stressing the things the person can still do and enjoy. Most people want to help and support you; let them know exactly how they can do it. ***Stress the positives***. Here are some examples:

- "Grandma loves to tell stories about growing up on the farm. Sometimes the stories may sound mixed up. Listen to her and ask questions even if the answers aren't right. This makes her happy."

- "Dad is likely to ask you the same questions over and over. Answer him like it's the first time he asked you. Please don't argue with him about things that don't matter."

- "Mary loves to go out to dinner. She struggles with reading the menu. Please help her to make a choice and please include her in the conversation."

- "Grandpa always enjoyed drinking a beer (or two) at dinnertime. But now he gets confused when he drinks alcohol. Feel free to bring along a non-alcoholic beer and offer it to him. He will love that!"

- "Mom no longer cooks, and I am not a very good one. We love to eat and would appreciate you cooking or bringing in a meal during your visit."

TIP #7: Give family and friends tips on how they can communicate with your person

Communication changes throughout the course of the illness. Yet, successful communication is possible when we consider the following:

- Call the person by their preferred name (for many it is a nickname). This may seem weird but, if they don't remember being a grandma, they may not respond to you when you greet them by saying, "Hi Grandma."

- Be sure to get their attention when you are talking. Your person is now much more distractible. Turn off the TV or radio if it interferes with conversation.

- Always include your person in the conversation. Don't talk past him like he is not present.

- Slow down and make sure she understands what you are saying.

- When you ask a question, give him time to respond (it could be up to 20 seconds or more).

- If you see her struggling, offer a guess or let her know it's okay – she can tell you later.

- Don't correct him if his answer is wrong. If there is no harm in what he is saying, just go along with it and then gently try to change the subject.

- Don't argue! This is one battle you will not win. Let the subject go.

- Don't ask a "yes or no" question if you are not willing to take "no" for an answer. Otherwise, you will begin to explain, reason, convince or coerce someone who has already told you "NO!" This **will** result in an unwanted argument. Let it go and try again later.

- A simple statement may be easier than a question. Instead of asking, "Do you want to use the restroom?" say, "Let's use the restroom before we leave."

- Watch your body language, facial expressions, and tone of voice. This is 93% of your message4. If your person sees or hears upset in your face or voice, he will also quickly become upset. However, if he sees a soft, warm smile and hears a calm voice, he will respond accordingly.

- Always remember, she is a dignified adult. There is no need to talk or treat her like she is a child who does not understand.

TIP #8: Be sure to factor in rest periods throughout the day

Fatigue, fatigue, fatigue. As I've stressed, again and again, fatigue is the enemy of the human brain – especially for those living with dementia. Rest can restore the ability to function and will improve mood as well.

Be sure you know what fatigue looks like in your person. For many, it looks like greater confusion, irritability, speaking out of turn, becoming quiet, or looking spaced out. Do not expect your person to initiate the rest period (especially when this has been a person who never rested). Instead, invite them to join you for a glass of lemonade on the deck; watch a favorite TV sitcom or sport; look at

---

4   Mehrabian, A., & Wiener, M. (1967). Decoding of inconsistent communications. *Journal of Personality and Social Psychology, 6*(1), 109-114.

the newspaper or cruise itinerary; etc. Try to promote a 30-minute quiet time, a couple of times during the day.

Naps can be very refreshing. Even a late afternoon nap can help minimize evening confusion. Perhaps you can initiate the nap by saying, "We're on vacation. Let's treat ourselves to a nap!" Be aware that when the person naps in bed, they may think it is morning when they wake. Since you are on vacation, take your time to reorient them to the day. Say things like, "We had such a good nap. I think I worked up an appetite for dinner!" Most importantly, just keep the day moving forward; your person can catch up (if that is even important).

TIP #9: On bad days, prepare yourself, family and friends for Plan B

Many of us notice that during a trip there are days that we wake up and wish we could just relax instead of heading out for another scheduled activity. Just as you have educated your family and friends about your person's condition, routine, and best communication skills, make sure they stay flexible and supportive of whatever you and your person need to make this trip successful.

Give yourself permission to sit out activities. Look at the trip as a marathon, not a sprint. Passing on an activity or two may mean greater success throughout the trip.

Imagine your son and his family are staying with you and they have tickets to see a spring training game with you and your wife with dementia. They see that she is having a bad morning, but she is insisting on going to the game. Help your son and his family to make an excuse to leave and come back after the game. Or better yet, ask one of the grandchildren to stay behind and take Grandma to lunch, so you can enjoy the game with your family. Let the grandchild know how to keep Grandma engaged during the day.

TIP #10: If there is growing confusion and restlessness, it's okay to cut the trip short

As you've learned, having a backup plan is essential. You have factored in all the things it will take to make this a successful trip. But even with good planning and support of family and friends, the person may not be able to adapt and can become restless, irritable, confused or demand to go home. Do not take this as a failure on your part. You did your best. Rather, see this as another change in your person's condition. Focus on getting home and back into your routine.

If family or friends are staying with you and observe growing restlessness and confusion, kindly ask them if they would adjust their plans for the rest of the trip. Remind them that this is not an indication of how either you or your loved one feels about them; rather it is an indication that your person has become fatigued and overwhelmed.

Summer Escape Abandoned!

Jim and Lori relocated from North Dakota to Arizona following her diagnosis of Lewy Body Disease. They both agreed it would be helpful to live closer to their adult daughter. However, the summers were hot, so Jim decided that they would rent a summer home in the mountains. Lori was in favor of this plan and the couple set off for a planned three-month stay.

About a week into the trip, Lori announced that "a man came by looking for a nice home to rent." She conveyed to Jim that she had agreed to show the man the summer home and that they would return to their home in Phoenix. Jim initially tried to explain to Lori that they had paid for the home and they would stay on for several more months. However, it was very clear to Jim that Lori did not understand this as she became adamant that the "man will be coming by in the afternoon to look at the place."

Jim was aware that she often had delusions and the best thing he could do was to go along with her ideas. The couple patiently waited one afternoon, and then the next, for the man to arrive. Of course, no man ever showed up, but Lori's false belief continued. Jim took this as his clue to return to their home in Phoenix rather than trying to get her to stay longer in a home that created more confusion for her.

The couple returned home, and Lori never spoke of the man again. Jim considered this a great lesson about Lori's ability to travel from the comfort of their home.

CHAPTER 8

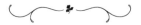

10 Essential Documents to Carry When You Travel

Trip preparation also includes ensuring that you have all the necessary documents you may need along the way. Ideally, these documents have already been gathered for daily life and in case of an emergency.

Many caregivers try to assemble a summary sheet of important documents to have available should a sudden health issue strike their loved one or themselves. If you have such a list, you will be able to pull together travel documents much more quickly.

DOCUMENT 1: Identification Cards

Having a valid identification card is essential for travel. For domestic travel, a driver's license or travel ID will be needed. Beginning October 1, 2020, a Real ID will be required for travel. (Visit your state's driver's licensing agency website to find out exactly what documentation is required to obtain a REAL ID.)

Since many people living with dementia may no longer have a valid driver's license, it is best to contact your local Department of Motor Vehicles to determine how to obtain a valid travel ID for your person. For those who are homebound, some states will have a field agent who may come to your home to take a picture and complete the paperwork. Some families have also used a traveling notary to assist with the process.

Foreign travel will require a current passport. For those who already have a passport, simply get an updated picture and apply online for a new one.

Now that you have the needed identification card(s), it is essential to **make copies** to carry with you, should the ID be lost or forgotten at a checkpoint along the way. Another option is to take a picture of the ID and keep it on your cell phone or in the cloud. Thus, it is a good idea to get WiFi wherever you travel to ensure access to this information.

It is not uncommon for many travelers to leave or misplace their IDs, wallets, cellphones, etc., in security lines, hotels, or restaurants. There is nothing worse than getting to the airport and finding your person does not have an ID. ***Look for ID at least one day before you travel***.

TSA (the U.S. Transportation Security Administration) will allow people to travel without a travel ID. **However**, the passenger will need to show up at least two hours in advance to complete an identity verification process. That process includes collecting information such as your name, current address, and other personal information that will confirm their identity. Having other forms of ID, including a social security card, credit card or even a Costco card, will provide added information about your person. (For more information, please visit www.tsa.gov.)

While most people in the early stages of dementia will be able to carry their own ID, it is best that – throughout the trip – their traveling companion ensures ID is safely returned to a wallet or purse whenever it has been presented. This is especially true with security checkpoints and when using credit cards during retail or restaurant transactions.

Be sure to carry a current picture of your person should you get separated and need to contact the authorities. During a support group meeting, one caregiver shared that when traveling with her husband, she took a picture of him each day so she could also provide information as to what he was wearing.

DOCUMENT 2: Medication List

Most seasoned travelers understand that it is essential to carry medications on their person during travel, should bags get lost or travel become delayed. It is also wise to bring an extra three-day supply, to work around unexpected issues.

Carrying an updated **medication list** will aid the traveler should more medication be needed during travel. If the individual becomes ill during while traveling, a medical provider will ask about any routine or 'as needed' medications.

It is best to record:

- **Name of medication(s), dosage, and frequency taken.**
  Include both the trade and generic names. (If you are traveling outside of the U.S., most medications are recognized by generic label.) Include over-the-counter and as-needed medications as well.

- **Name and phone number of the pharmacy dispensing the medication**.

- **Name and phone number of the medical provider** who prescribed the medication.

- **Include a list of allergies** to medication, food or any other known allergies.

Table 3

Table 3 shows an example of a medication list:

Table 3. Sample Medication List				
Name: Sue Jones Allergies: Penicillin, latex, strawberries				
Medication name	Dosage & Frequency	Reason	Pharmacy Information	Medical Provider Information
Aricept/donepezil	10 mg; every night	Alzheimer's disease	CVS, 212-222-2222	Dr. Michael Smith (neurologist) 212-223-3333
Zestril/lisinopril	10 mg; every morning	High blood pressure	CVS, 212-222-2222	Dr. Allison Brown (family doctor) 212-223-4444
Melatonin	5 mg; bedtime	Sleep	Over-the-counter	Self-prescribed
Zyrtec/Cetirizine	10 mg; daily as need	Seasonal allergies	Over-the-counter	Dr. Allison Brown 212-223-4444

DOCUMENT 3: List of Health Conditions/Medical Providers

This list should provide general information about more serious physical and mental conditions and any helpful medical history. For example, diabetes, dementia, and past cardiovascular and cerebrovascular events (with dates) is important information to include. Include the **active** medical provider's name and contact number for each of the conditions.

DOCUMENT 4: Medical Documents

Many individuals living with dementia will also have identified 'agents' who have been appointed or named by the person to make medical and/or financial decisions on their behalf. These individuals have what is often referred to as **Power of Attorney**. Some individuals may also have a court-appointed guardian or conservator. In general, the guardian will make medical decisions on the person's behalf while the conservator can make financial decisions.

Plan to bring copies of relevant Power of Attorney or guardianship forms and documents. With growing health privacy laws, many healthcare institutions will ask you for these documents before sharing medical information with you or allowing you to make decisions on your person's behalf.

If you or your person have stated health care wishes, including Do Not Resuscitate (DNR), Living Will, or other forms naming specific health care decisions, be sure to include a copy of the state-sponsored and physician-signed DNR order or Physician Orders for Life-Sustaining Treatment (POLST) form. This is most important for those with advancing dementia. Note that some states have online registries allowing electronic storage and access your medical directives. Check with your state about this option.

DOCUMENT 5: Insurance Cards and/or Travel/Medical Insurance

Include copies of all up-to-date insurance cards, including Medicare, Medicaid, commercial and/or supplemental plans. This information can help ensure that you or your person's medical care is billed correctly from the start, even if the original cards are left behind in the rush to the hospital or clinic.

For older travelers or those with chronic or serious health issues, **_travel insurance_** can provide additional peace of mind. Travel insurance not only provides trip protection, should the trip need to be cancelled, but can also defray additional costs should an unplanned health issue occur. The policy may offer reimbursement for medical expenses and can also cover the cost of medical evacuation, avoiding an out-of-pocket expense for you or your person. As you plan your travels, it is essential to consult with a travel agent about the best options available.

DOCUMENT 6: 'In Case of Emergency' Numbers

During times of stress and crisis, the ability to remember important phone numbers will be taxed. It is important to carry a list of contact information that you can use, or give to another person to use, should an urgent situation arise.

In addition to immediate family members, you may also want to include the house sitter, kennel (if boarding animals), and close friends. For each emergency contact, be sure to list:

- The contact's name.

- Their relationship to you and/or your person, and

- Preferred contact numbers.

DOCUMENT 7: Credit Card Information

It is not uncommon for a credit or debit card to be lost, stolen or compromised during travel. That's why it is important to create a list of each of the credit and debit cards you will use during your trip. ***The list must include:***

- The type of card.

- The card number.

- The name of the issuing bank.

- The 800 number to call in an emergency.

As with other travel documents, you may also want to take a photo of each credit card. Remember to store all this information safely – don't leave it in a hotel room drawer or any other spot that may be accessible to people you don't know.

While in the past you may each have traveled with a separate card, you may want to determine whether your person is still able to manage that responsibility.

It is essential to notify the bank of any foreign travel, so your bank does not disable your card for fear of fraud. When in doubt, contact your credit card company in advance of travel.

DOCUMENT 8: Travel Documents/Travel Agent Contact Information

These days, the travel industry digitizes most travel documents. However, you may find it helpful to print and carry your travel documents with you. Many travelers choose to organize their documents in a binder, sorted by day or by travel type (i.e., airline, rental car, hotel, etc.).

If you used a travel agent, be sure to carry their name, phone number and/or email so they can assist you if needed documents are lost. In addition, carry the phone numbers for any other travel or excursion plans that involve a reservation.

For example, let's imagine you are on a road trip and have a reservation at a hotel that is 250 miles away. You need to make an unplanned stop and stayover somewhere else because your person is becoming more confused. The ease of having that travel information at your fingertips will minimize the added stress you might feel while making new arrangements.

DOCUMENT 9: Itinerary

Having a written or printed itinerary can be helpful, especially since we all tend to lose track of dates during a longer trip. Although many travel agents, cruises, and group travel tours will provide an itinerary, they're almost always electronic. ***Ask for paper copies or plan to print your own copies.***

Even if you're planning your own trip – perhaps a visit with family and friends – a written itinerary can prove to be quite useful.

Most importantly, ***share your itinerary with your emergency contacts*** so they know where you are and how to get in contact with you. You will want to include:

- Departure and return dates (flight/train/driving plans).

- Planned stays throughout the trip, including phone numbers for hotels, or for the homes of family or friends.

- Emergency contact information if you'll be at sea or traveling outside the country.

DOCUMENT 10: Companion Card

Respect and dignity are at the core of caring for and/or traveling with a person living with dementia.

You have read how the demands of travel can lead to unwanted behaviors as the person becomes fatigued, overwhelmed, confused and/or frustrated. Keep in mind that others may not know or understand that your person has dementia. They also will not know how to respond in a way that is helpful for you and your person.

The companion card (Please see Chapter 1, Sample 1: Companion Card) provides a discrete and respectful way to let others know your person is having a difficult time. Companion cards are the size of a business card and can be carried in your wallet, purse, or pocket. You may want to order a box of them to have available for your use and to provide to other family caregivers.

Here are some examples that show how you might use a companion card:

- Perhaps you are flying on a plane and your person becomes very anxious and restless and is seated in the center. The passenger next to your person does not understand what is happening. By providing the companion card to the adjacent passenger, you're offering them the opportunity to be more patient with your person.

- Or, maybe you are eating at a restaurant and your father is very rude to the wait staff. Once again, providing the companion card can help to defuse a stressful situation.

You can also provide the companion card as you go through security lines, giving the agents a chance to be more alert and attentive to various medical conditions. The TSA also provides a printable 'TSA Notification Card' (Find it at www.tsa.gov) that allows the traveler to write-in the medical condition or disability to alert TSA staff.

CHAPTER 9

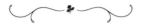

10 Tips for Keeping Your Person Occupied during Travel

With your person's lost sense of time and what might seem to be an eternally long trip to both of you, it is best to plan for how you will keep your person meaningfully engaged and occupied. This will be especially helpful to avoid any anxiety that might occur during delays or even on a long day.

TIP #1: Think about the things that your person enjoys doing at home, either alone or with you

Make a list of these activities so you can use them during travel. For many, this includes reading (or looking through) a favorite magazine or newspaper, watching a familiar TV show or movie, listening to music, enjoying a snack, or even trying a new game or activity.

Table 4

Here, in Table 4, is a list of activities. ***Use it to build your own list and to create a travel bag of activities for your person:***

Table 4: Travel Activities	
Simple games: - Deck of cards - Domino set Puzzles/word games: - Large font word search - Large font crossword puzzle - Simple maze games Reading material: - Favorite and familiar newspapers - Favorite and familiar magazines - Magazines/books with favorite images - Reminisce Magazine (www.reminisce.com) - Short stories (e.g., Chicken Soup for the Soul) Audio: - Books on tape* - Playlist or music app(s) - Headphones - Split headphone jack	Computer/Tablet/Phone apps: - Familiar games - Painting images - Favorite TV shows, movies, sporting events Interactive: - Adult coloring books and colored pencils - Trivia games - Recording license plates Snacks: - Favorite finger foods (cookies, crackers, pretzels, etc.) - Fresh fruit - Favorite beverages (usually sweet)
* Note: with significant memory loss, your person may have a hard time following the plot.	

TIP #2: Purchase and prepare the activities you plan to bring along

Computer tablets, such as iPads, are very handy during travel to access email, business and travel documents. They also bring endless possibilities to keep your person (and you) occupied with a variety of games, music, TV shows, videos, and movies. If you don't know how to program your tablet with games, music or movies, ask a friend or a younger person to help you do so. (Some local libraries also offer assistance with technology related Apps and downloads.) Make sure you bring along a headset for your person to use, especially if you plan to play music or listen to a TV show or movie. You can also purchase a split headphone jack if you both want to listen in.

TIP #3: Music works for most

There is very clear research evidence that shows music has a profound positive impact on people living with dementia and can be enjoyed well into the late stages of the disease. Music can be calming, invigorating and memorable. These memories can transport us back to a time and place that can be very comforting, especially for the person living with dementia.

Make a playlist of favorite music for your person. If you don't know your person's preferred music or genre, consider looking for music that was most popular during the time that person was 18 to 25 years of age. You can do an internet search for popular music by year that will help you hone in on the favorites your person may enjoy.

If making a playlist seems like a daunting task, there are also numerous music apps such as Pandora, Spotify, and others that not only focus on a specific genre, but also allow you to listen to the most popular music by decade or artist. These services usually have a small subscription fee. Be sure to purchase the app for your phone or tablet well before the trip and try it out with your person. When Wi-Fi is available, these can be handy to use. Note that some of these apps will also allow you to create your own playlist in advance, to listen in when Wi-Fi is not available.

TIP #4: Prepare a carry-on bag that will include the items you plan to use

As the old adage reminds us, "Variety is the spice of life!" Be sure you have a variety of things you can use during your trip. Many of the props – electronic tablet, games, magazines, and snacks – you will need are compact, so it is better to bring too many along than not enough. (Use Table 4 to help you assemble a travel bag that works for your person.)

These same activities can be used during group excursions or activities as you observe your person becoming restless. Be sure to bring your bag of activities wherever you go. You just never know when it will come in handy.

Don't worry too much about repetition. One advantage, for those living with memory loss, is that they will rapidly forget that they participated in a recent activity. So, when you suggest looking at the newspaper (again), the person may be happy to take a look, having forgotten he just looked at it 30 minutes ago.

TIP #5: Offer these activities one at a time, inviting the person to engage with you

It is not uncommon for people living with dementia to have difficulty initiating an activity. Your assistance in choosing an activity can help. For example, during your flight, you can pull out your tablet and headphones and say to your person, "Let's watch 'I Love Lucy'!" and begin to play an episode or two. Your activity suggestion can relieve the stress on both of you.

Or, perhaps you'd like to sit out by the adult pool on the cruise ship, but you think your wife will get restless. You bring along an adult coloring book and pencils and ask her to help you out. Now, she becomes engaged in coloring and soon she is working on a piece of art while you enjoy a brief break and read a book.

TIP #6: Make sure that other travel companions know how to engage your person

If you are traveling with other family and friends, they, too, can help keep your person engaged. Whether through interesting conversations, enjoying a magazine or listening to music together, your travel companions will probably need you to tell them what to do and show them what works. Don't be afraid to ask them to help.

TIP #7: Watch for signs of fatigue or frustration and be prepared to stop when you observe either

Hopefully, you have determined, well before your trip, what games and activities your person likes and can feel successful with, even if they don't do it correctly.

At the same time, be aware that fatigue can keep your person from engaging in those pre-planned pastimes in a meaningful way which may lead to frustration. During times of fatigue, try listening to favorite quiet music or looking at calming images (for example, landscapes, water, or food) in a book or magazine. Doing nothing is also an option. Encourage rest or a nap if that seems feasible.

Regardless of the cause, simply and gently end the activity and offer another distraction such as a piece of chocolate.

TIP #8: Find a pleasant way to end the activity

Transitioning from one activity to another can take time, patience, and finesse, particularly if your person is engrossed in what they are doing. Try suggesting a new activity, sharing a snack or taking a walk.

Always be respectful when negotiating these changes. Your person is not a child.

TIP #9: Bring your own snacks

You know what snacks and beverages your person likes, so having them readily available can be very helpful. During travel, carry enough for the day or outing, and keep a stock in your room for ready access. By having these favorites on-hand, you don't have to wait on flight attendants, slow service in a restaurant or during unexpected delays. Don't be surprised if most of the desired snacks are sweet, as most people living with dementia will develop a tendency to want to eat food that is sweet in flavor and soft in texture. Besides, special treats are part of most everyone's travel experience.

TIP #10: Be creative and use the experiences around you

Sometimes, the best props for engagement are right under our noses. For example, cruise ships are often full of beautiful art in the hallways, dining rooms, lounges, and other areas. Many also sell art while at sea, offering an opportunity for your person to view and enjoy them.

Perhaps you are part of a tour group visiting an art museum. If he cannot join in a very long and dry discussion, perhaps you take him to a single painting and begin asking questions like:

- "What do you think of this picture?"

- "What color stands out most to you?"

- "How does this picture make you feel?"

- "Would you want to buy this picture?"

- "How much would you pay for it?"

- "Where would you hang it in your house?"

Or, maybe you are taking a long day trip in the car or on a bus. You could engage your person in a discussion with questions like:

- "Where do you think all these people are going?"

- "Shall we see how many blue cars we can spot in the next five minutes?"

- "Do you remember when we took the kids on a trip to Disneyland?"

Here's another scenario: you're out for dinner and your person becomes impatient waiting on their food. Can you become observers of other diners by asking your person:

- "Do you think anyone here is celebrating a birthday tonight?"

- "What kind of birthday cake do you think they will serve here?"

- "Did you see the cute little girl with her mom? That reminds me of when our daughter was young."

You get the idea – be creative. Get your person talking and make it fun and interesting. The goal here is to keep your person occupied in a meaningful way.

Got Diversions?

Suzy is a registered nurse who was hired by a family to assist them and accompany their dad, Bob, from his home in Indiana to his new home, an assisted living community in California.

Suzy learned Bob had vascular dementia, along with difficulty with speech. He could be quite impulsive and needed close supervision for toileting and eating.

Because Suzy was aware that this would be a six-hour trip with a connection in Atlanta, she took time to learn Bob's favorite foods, along with activities she could use to keep him occupied during this long trip.

Equipped with a well-stocked backpack, Suzy's hands were free at all times to assist Bob while at the airport. She engaged Bob in several short TV programs that she had on her tablet. She asked him to sort a deck of cards for her and then engaged him in a game of Fish. Together, they worked on a game of Solitaire. They colored pictures of fish as she reminisced with him about his fishing adventures. She was glad she brought plenty of his favorite candy along since there was a delay with their connecting flight to California.

On the connecting flight, Suzy used the same diversion tactics to keep Bob occupied and comfortable. She accompanied him to the toilet and, later, made sure he enjoyed his favorite beverage – cranberry juice. After ten hours of travel, they arrived at their destination. Bob was clearly fatigued, but with Suzy's help and many great diversions, he tolerated the trip to his new home.

CHAPTER 10

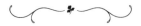

10 Tips for Safely Using 'As Needed' Medications during Travel

Daily routines are typically disrupted during travel. Combined with the challenges of managing the changing concept of time, along with planning and problem-solving, it is not uncommon for many individuals living with dementia to become more anxious before or during travel.

Your person's sleep may also be compromised when she is away from the comfort and familiarity of home. As we noted earlier in Chapter 5 (10 Reasons to Avoid or Reconsider Travel), for individuals living with dementia who are easily prone to upset, physical restlessness, verbal outbursts or psychosis, it may be best not to travel. However, sometimes travel might become necessary, along with the use of 'as needed' medications prescribed by the medical provider.

Here are some important tips and considerations about using "as needed" (also known as 'PRN') medications:

TIP #1: Meet with the person's medical provider well in advance of travel

Several weeks prior to travel, it is best to visit with your person's medical provider to discuss the upcoming travel and determine the best way to manage symptoms. Some emotional and/or behavioral symptoms may warrant routine use of already-prescribed medications. However, during travel, sometimes 'as needed' medications may be prescribed, as well.

The range of potential new symptoms is wide. Many people living with dementia already experience periodic difficulties with emotions and behavioral expressions during the course of the illness. Anxiety and depression can be quite common as people lose the ability to plan and problem solve. Some appear to lack interest as they start to have difficulty beginning or even engaging in a favorite activity. Travel can trigger or exaggerate these kinds of symptoms.

For some, this can result in some sleeping throughout most of the day, making sleep at night more challenging. Likewise, those with hallucinations, delusions or paranoid thoughts can be more edgy, particularly if any of these symptoms are persistent and upsetting to the person.

If you or other family caregivers observe any of these changes, be sure they are reported to the medical provider for further assessment and treatment considerations.

TIP #2: Be specific about the symptoms you are observing in your person

As you meet with your person's medical provider before you go, be very honest and specific about what your person is experiencing. Let them know what you are hoping to achieve by reporting this problem. Here are examples of specific symptom descriptions:

- "He becomes very anxious when I am out of his sight."

- "She is sleeping six to eight hours during the day and wants to go to bed by 7:00 p.m. but then gets me up at 4:00 a.m."

- "She gets easily overwhelmed and often begins to cry."

- "He becomes very angry and rude when we go out to eat and he has to wait for his food to come."

- "Every afternoon around 4:00 p.m., he starts pacing about the house, becomes more physically restless and is prone to outbursts when I ask him to sit down."

If a medication is prescribed for emotional, behavioral or sleep issues, the medical provider should help you understand what benefit(s) the medication may provide and how long it takes before it begins to act.

TIP #3: Discuss other ways to problem-solve beyond medication

Sometimes instead of – or in addition to – a medication, a non-medication intervention should be considered. For example, for the person sleeping throughout the day and up very early in the morning, keeping her active and involved in an Adult Day Health Care program may assist with better sleep at night. Or, by watching a pre-recorded TV show, listening to music, or playing a game, you may be able to keep her up later in the evening, thus helping her sleep later in the morning.

For the person who becomes impatient while waiting for food, bringing a favorite snack along or ordering an appetizer before the meal may be enough to help him better manage his emotions. These are just a few examples of learning and applying new problem-solving techniques.

The Alzheimer's Association provides many quick tips for family caregivers and travel companions to respond to various types of upset. Visit www.alz.org and search "behaviors."

TIP #4: Try out medication in advance of travel

Every person responds to medication differently. Some medications may take weeks before the desired effect is seen. Others may be quick-acting with benefits seen in 30 minutes to one hour.

It is important to understand how your person will respond to any new medication or increased dose or strength of an already-prescribed medication. Even 'as needed' medication should be tried out well before your trip.

TIP #5: Carefully watch for any benefit or unwanted side effects

Sometimes the medication prescribed has an opposite effect than what was anticipated or has other unwanted side effects. For example, an 'as needed' medication might be prescribed for anxiety during travel; but when given, the person becomes even more anxious. If your person experiences any negative side effects, notify the prescribing medical provider immediately. There may be other options available.

TIP #6: Learn how long it takes before medication works

Some medications used for emotional or behavioral issues work best when given regularly. Other medications may work better when given on a limited basis, only to manage the symptom that has been identified. To set reasonable expectations about how medications may or may not benefit your person's symptoms, ask clear questions of the prescribing medical provider.

TIP #7: Be aware of certain over-the-counter medications

Believe it or not, some over-the-counter (OTC) medications can have serious and unwanted side effects in older adults. However, because they are available without a prescription, many of us think they are safe for everyone.

Many people who have difficulty with sleep will turn to OTC sleep aids that contain an ingredient called *diphenhydramine*. Unfortunately, the chemical properties of this compound can cause increased confusion in older people (even those without dementia). Diphenhydramine is also contained in many antihistamines used for colds and allergies and can be sometimes be found in medications to help with motion sickness.

Another caution for older adults is the use of OTC pain medications. Tylenol (acetaminophen) is by far the safest of the OTC pain options. Pain medications classified as NSAIDs (non-steroidal anti-inflammatory drugs) like ibuprofen and naproxen should be used cautiously in older adults. These medications can increase the risk of bleeding of the stomach and/or bowels; decrease kidney function; interfere with blood pressure medication, and; cause fluid retention that can increase the risk of heart failure.

TIP #8: Use your pharmacist as your expert

It is important that your medical providers know of any OTC medications your person takes, either routinely or 'as needed.' Likewise, your local pharmacist is a great resource in guiding your choice of OTC medications, especially when combined with prescribed 'as needed' or routine medications. Don't hesitate to consult with pharmacists with any medication-related questions you may have.

TIP #9: Consider taking along other OTC medication/products

Since you will probably visit your local pharmacy to get medications filled before your trip, take a moment to purchase other products that you may need during travel. These could range from hand sanitizer to OTC medications to help manage other unexpected physical symptoms that occur.

Consider bringing along the following:

- Antacids like Tums®.

- Mild laxatives like Dulcolax®.

- Pain relievers like Tylenol® or generic acetaminophen.

- Cold medication (make sure it does **not** contain diphenhydramine).

- Cough drops.

- Eye drops and/or saline solution.

- Sunscreen.

- Hand sanitizer or wipes.

As mentioned above, remember to consult your pharmacist for any questions you may have about the use of these products in combination with any other oral or topical medication(s) that have been prescribed for your person.

TIP #10: Consider taking first aid products

Depending on where you plan to travel, it never hurts to come prepared with a few extra items in case of a bump, bruise, cut or insect bite! Consider packing Band-Aids, disinfectant wipes, elastic wraps, support hose (for long flights or prolonged sitting), antibiotic ointment, bug repellant, and calamine lotion to soothe burns.

A small flashlight can also be helpful in case of a power outage or if you or your person needs to go outside at night. A little preparation will save you a last-minute trip to the local pharmacy.

CHAPTER 11

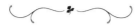

10 Tips to Assist with Personal Care

As people living with dementia progress into the middle or moderate stage of the condition, they will need assistance with personal care activities such as grooming, bathing, dressing, toileting, and eating. While some will need gentle reminders, others will need more specific directions and cues, or, in many cases, hands-on assistance. (*Please see Chapter 1, Table 1, Stages of Dementia.*)

When travel takes a person away from the familiarity of home, families often report there is more confusion around these daily activities. It can take you and your family by surprise because, at home, very little support has been needed.

A calm and dignified approach while traveling will help you assist your person to look their very best during the trip. Remember, ***the goal is not perfection***. While in the past, your mom might have coordinated her jewelry, shoes, and handbag with her clothing, the goal now is to be patient and help her look and feel her best, just for today.

Use these added tips to make personal care more successful:

TIP #1: Use the daily routine to prompt personal care activities

We all rely on daily routines – they are the rituals that keep us comfortable. As you prepare to travel as a caregiver, be sure to factor in your loved one's personal care routines, as well.

If your person likes to have breakfast before dressing for the day, it will be important to honor this preference. If staying with family or friends, let your hosts know that your wife will be coming to breakfast in her robe. If in a hotel or on a cruise, order room service or provide the most presentable option for her to go down to the breakfast area.

One of the best approaches is to use routines and habits to guide your person. Imagine your husband needs to take a shower due to body odor, but he is refusing. You know he likes to shower before going to church. In this situation, prompt him by saying, "We are going to church. I know you like to get cleaned up before we go. Let's get started!" Remember, you don't need to be going to church and he will probably forget; but now he is bathed, comfortable and dignified. And, as a bonus, you did **not** have to argue about it.

Missing Bath

Cindy and Dan accompanied Dan's parents on a dream trip to Ireland. Before leaving on the trip, Cindy began to have some concerns about her mother-in-law's changing memory.

Over the two-week trip, she observed her mother-in-law's hygiene was slipping. Her hair was often uncombed and unwashed, and Cindy noted growing body odor.

Cindy discretely inquired with her father-in-law to see if she might be able to assist her mother-in-law with grooming tasks. He noted the room had only a shower, which was a problem since Mom always took baths at home. To make matters worse, no washcloths were available in the room. The combined effect made Mom's confusion worse as she was unable to get herself cleaned up.

Cindy tried, very gently, to assist her mother-in-law but all attempts were met with resistance. Together, Cindy, Dan, and her father-in-law decided not to cause upset by making an issue of it. However, they realized it was time to consult with a medical provider upon return and for the next trip, they would need to think through these challenges well ahead of time.

TIP #2: Bring familiar products from home and lay them out for the person to see

With the loss of reading comprehension, seeing a familiar product used at home will make it much easier for your person to complete grooming and bathing. When traveling, bring the favorite shampoo and soap with you. The ones provided by the hotel or host family will look unfamiliar and will probably go unused.

Since bathing is one of the most overwhelming tasks your person deals with, it helps to think ahead and lay out the items that will prompt and support your person with hygiene activities. When it's time for your person to clean up, have the bath or shower ready to go with clean clothes laid out and ready to put on, once bathing is finished.

TIP #3: Positively direct your person through these activities, giving instructions for each step as needed

Avoid asking your person, "Have you taken your shower?" or "Would you like to brush your teeth now?" You are likely to hear, "I've already taken a shower," and "No, I will brush my teeth later." You asked the question because you wanted to prompt the activity; yet, now, you may feel like you need to correct, coerce, or convince your loved to do what you've asked. They already told you, "No!" An argument is on its way and you are about to lose!

Instead, direct them in a positive way by saying, "Let's get ready for the day," or "Why don't we freshen up before we meet the kids for breakfast?" Perhaps you can gently take your person by the hand and lead them to the bathroom.

Most daily activities include multiple steps. Sometimes, all you need to do is to get the activity started – for example, initiate hair brushing by handing your person a brush.

In other cases, multiple-step activities may require specific instructions for each part of the activity. For example, when helping Mom put on her makeup, you may want to hand her the single product she needs before moving onto the next step. By observing and planning the activity in advance, you can break it into several steps and make life a little easier.

TIP #4: Adapt rather than argue

Sometimes, no matter what activity you request, you'll be met with resistance. For example, as we've seen, if your person **believes** they've already bathed, they're quite likely to refuse.

Instead of arguing, think about how you might adapt the situation to get your person as clean as possible before going out for the day. Could you assist with a sponge bath by filling the sink with warm water and some no-rinse soap? Could you use wet wipes or a warm washcloth to clean the essential parts?

For the person who insists on wearing the same clothing, think about purchasing and bringing along multiple items that look the same. It could be that one particular shirt and one pair of pants are the only things your person recognizes as clothing. Duplicates can solve that problem.

Can't get the teeth brushed? Provide mouthwash or breath mints during the day and try again later.

The more flexible you are, the more likely the activity will get completed during the trip.

TIP #5: Don't rush your person as they are getting ready

You've probably noticed by now that it takes much longer than in the past for your person to get ready to go or to complete even simple tasks. **Rushing your loved one will add more pressure and likely slow things down as they try hard to hurry up.** With their lost sense of time, your reminders will add to the feelings of overwhelm and frustration. And, your added impatience is probably showing, making things worse.

Pay attention to how much time it actually takes for your person to get ready in the morning, eat meals or engage in other daily activities. **Factor that into your plans and let others know.** If your person can't be ready early in the morning, then kindly turn down early morning invitations and appointments. If your person needs a full hour to eat lunch, schedule accordingly.

Just remember, it will take longer to complete tasks, especially when in a new location.

TIP #6: Offer choices whenever feasible

People living with dementia want to maintain independence and normalcy for as long as possible. While simplifying tasks and choices can be helpful, stripping them away entirely will cause greater dependence, far earlier than necessary.

Consider this: we all give thought to what we will wear each day, based upon our plans for the day and weather conditions. Yet, your loved one may not think through these considerations.

Imagine you are on a cruise ship that is cold, but you plan to walk along the beach during a short excursion. You know to wear a sweater that you can take off and put in your bag; but your loved one is cold and dresses in slacks, a turtleneck sweater, and jacket. Now, you're in the unfortunate position of having to try to get her to understand that you're going to the beach and she is not prepared. In this case, a simple statement of choice would be better: "Mom, we are going to the beach this morning. Would you like to wear the pink or blue shirt with your shorts? And, why don't we bring a sweater along?" Now, she understands what is happening and can participate in making a decision.

Eating is another example of a time when choices need to be presented and supported. (*Please refer to Chapter 13, 10 Tips for Dining Out.*)

Factor in choice whenever you can. Your loved one is an adult and wants to feel included in decisions when possible.

TIP #7: Gently initiate the activity or let your person watch you perform the activity

Many of our daily activities are based on motor memory. Once we get going, we don't have to consciously think about what we are doing. When you brush your teeth, wash your hair in the shower or shave, you do it the same way every time, knowing exactly which products to use, and how to initiate and follow through to complete the task.

As dementia progresses, sometimes the verbal prompts don't make sense, or the person gets mixed up when carrying out an activity. In these situations, your gentle prompting, using visual or physical cues, can be most helpful. Get your loved one to the room where the activity needs to occur. Perhaps seeing the toothbrush laying out on the bathroom sink with toothpaste on it will prompt them to brush their teeth. Maybe your person needs you to put the toothbrush in his hand, slowly bring it up to his mouth and begin moving the toothbrush back and forth. Or perhaps you can brush your teeth together as he watches you in the mirror.

In general, these routine, repetitive activities can be maintained much longer when we support them with respectful and relaxed approaches.

TIP #8: Utilize the services of a hairdresser, barber or spa

Many families report that getting their person to wash hair can be challenging at home **and** during travel. Think about the added service that a hairstylist or barber can provide. Your person's social behavior will appear and you are likely to see them be very cooperative as hair is washed and styled, or while they get a good shave.

Consider using spa services on a cruise or in a hotel. We all like to be pampered. Plus, it is now one less activity you need to worry about.

TIP #9: Provide positive feedback

We all feel best when we hear positive comments. Let your loved one know they're doing everything right. Tell him how handsome he looks today as you go out. Thank her for joining you at lunch. You get the idea – positive and sincere feedback works.

Avoid negative statements like, "You can't go out looking like that!" Instead say, "I love it when you wear that pretty pink dress. It makes your eyes shine. Please wear it for me tonight?"

TIP #10: Find the 'good enough'

Despite your best efforts, what happens – or doesn't happen – during care activities can be challenging. **Let go of perfection**. Your person is living with dementia and trying to do their very best. Our job is to support them in a dignified way.

Many family caregivers worry about being judged by family and friends about their person's appearance. Yet, these family and friends have no idea how challenging these tasks may have become for your loved one. As with other aspects of this condition, be sure to communicate openly about what is 'good enough.' Does it really matter if he comes to dinner with a soiled shirt, especially if he is happy and engages with the family during dinner? So what if the back of her hair is not combed? She is ready to go out on the short excursion with everyone!

Give yourself a break and find your 'good enough.'

CHAPTER 12

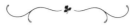

10 Tips for Managing Continence During Travel

Some people living with dementia may develop **incontinence**, the occasional loss of bladder and bowel control, as the disease progresses. Generally, it is because they no longer connect the physical signal that they **need** to go with the cognitive question of **where** to go.

The added stress of travel, change in routines, and unfamiliarity with where to find bathrooms can put your person traveling with dementia at greater risk for an incontinence episode. Sadly, to deal with the problem, some caregivers even resort to restricting fluid intake which can create more serious problems such as dehydration, constipation, and urinary tract infections.

A better approach is to employ some careful planning to successfully manage continence.

Here are some specific ways to do that:

TIP #1: Plan ahead and prompt toileting

Before leaving the house (ship, hotel, etc.), take a moment to locate restrooms at your destination for the day. Scouting out restrooms in airports, hotel lobbies, and highway exits will be essential. Then, by prompting use of a restroom every few hours, before meals and bedtime, you will assist in limiting accidents along the way. Even if your person tells you that they don't need to go, positively direct them to "try anyway, just in case we don't see a restroom again for a while." For those that need assistance with toileting, asking for family restrooms is most helpful.

TIP #2: Select practical clothing

Think ahead and identify dignified clothing choices that will also provide ease in using the toilet whether independently or with assistance. That means choosing pants that are easy to pull up and down and avoiding belts and buttons. (*Please see Resources: Dementia Specific Products Clothing.*)

TIP #3: Pack supplies you may need

When you find yourself concerned about not finding or getting to a toilet soon enough, or if your person has occasional incontinence episodes at home, plan to utilize an incontinence product during travel days. You will want to have extra products on hand during the trip and include a change of clothing if you think you'll need it.

TIP #4: Find the product that works best

Fortunately, advertisers and marketers who sell incontinence products have done us a favor; they are normalizing the idea that that many people can have incontinence issues and still live a full life without embarrassment. There are dozens of choices available to consumers and some companies will provide free samples to allow the consumer to find out what works best.

If your loved one has incontinence, think about which products will also make it easy for you to assist. For example, some products are easier to take on and off and can vary by absorbency. While pullups are easier for most, undergarments that fasten with Velcro or adhesive tabs are better for others. Some families find that for long haul air or road travel, using a nighttime product that is super absorbent along with an underpad on the seat provides the extra protection they are looking for. (*Please see Resources: Dementia Specific Products, Incontinence.*)

Even if your person has never had an incontinence episode, it still might be helpful to investigate in advance to find a product that might work.

TIP #5: Send products to your destination

If you don't have room in your luggage, or for those times when you can't find the particular product you use in a pharmacy, grocery or big box store, it is best to plan to ship the extra products ahead so you will have what you need along the way.

TIP #6: Fluids, fluids, fluids

For those with incontinence issues, there is a tendency to want to limit fluids. While this might be okay as you prepare for a three-hour flight, restricting fluids throughout the trip risks creating some of the more significant issues mentioned above: dehydration, constipation, urinary tract infection and/or increased confusion.

Ideally, water is the best choice to stay hydrated, but fruit juice, herbal tea, sports drinks, milk, ice cream, popsicles, and melons are also good choices. During your travel, be sure to offer a hydrating fluid throughout the day.

It's recommended that older adults should drink six to eight 8-ounce glasses of fluid per day. Yet, some people with dementia can become overwhelmed just by the size of the glass. Try using glassware that holds four to six ounces instead.

And remember that even though the glass may be sitting right by your person in the car, living room or restaurant, they may simply forget about it. Continue to encourage taking sips throughout the day.

Limit caffeinated products like coffee, energy drinks, and soda – they are not very hydrating and can stimulate the bladder! And keep alcohol to a minimum. Not only does it add to the confusion, but it is dehydrating as well.

Those with active bladders at night should get the bulk of their fluids in before 6 pm.

TIP #7: Plan for the nighttime

Most older adults are unable to sleep through the night without having to use the toilet at least once. Be sure to bring along night-lights or a pen light to make the bathroom easier to find and avoid a trip or fall.

Whether staying in a hotel room or on a cruise ship, ask to be placed in an accessible room that provides a toilet with a raised seat. Some families may even plan ahead to have a bedside commode available for ease of toileting at night.

If your loved one is prone to nighttime incontinence and the protective product leaks, plan to bring along extra pads, either washable or disposable. Ideally, you have tried these products before leaving home.

TIP #8: Use the toilet anyway

Even with the best continence products, it is important to use the toilet throughout the day. And, for those wearing continence products, the product should be changed following an incontinence episode to minimize the risk of developing a urinary tract infection.

TIP #9: Stay calm if an accident happens

Remember, it is truly an accident. You have prepared for this. Keep your emotions in check so your person won't feel embarrassed and refuse to participate in the trip.

TIP #10: Avoid constipation

From the change in routine to the changes in diet, dining hours, and fluid intake, we are all at risk for constipation during travel. One technique that works well is to simulate the travel routine at home, before your trip begins, to keep bowel movements regular.

We all benefit from taking in lots of hydrating fluids, eating a good breakfast and drinking a warm beverage in the morning. Plenty of fruits and vegetables provide the fiber needed. If your person typically takes over-the-counter products – from fiber to stool softeners to stimulants – plan to use those as needed during travel.

When the urge strikes, it is important to respond. Try to schedule additional time into the day when your person generally has a bowel movement (BM). You don't want to rush your loved one. If you do, you run the risk that they won't sit long enough and will become constipated.

Keep an eye out for regular BMs. If they are not happening, you may need to consider the use of an over-the-counter product. ***Don't let your person go more than three days without a BM.***

CHAPTER 13

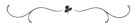

10 Tips for Hotel Stays

Home is the most comfortable and familiar place for the person living with dementia. Yet, even the poshest hotel may create some challenges for the person with dementia who wakes up in an unfamiliar setting.

There are certain amenities and room set-ups you can consider when booking a room, whether it's in a hotel, on a cruise ship or through a home-share service like Airbnb or VRBO (Vacation Rentals by Owner).

TIP #1: Think about the person's bedroom configuration at home

As humans, we operate using a lot of 'muscle memory.' When we wake during the night, we don't have to think about which way to look for the bedside clock or how to find the bathroom. Why not use your person's innate muscle memory to help them navigate a new location?

For example, on which side of the bed does your person usually sleep? Where is that space relative to the bathroom?

It will be much easier for the person living with dementia to locate the bathroom if they are approaching it from the same side as they do at home (that's an example of muscle memory in action). Try to create the 'props' that mimic your person's bedroom at home. Move a clock to their side of the bed. Place their usual glass of water by the bedside. These simple steps can help you and your person enjoy a more comfortable overnight stay.

TIP #2: Talk with the hotel directly

Compared to a booking agent or third-party website, hotel staff is much more likely to know the exact configuration of their rooms. Call ahead and explain the situation. And ask if they can reserve a room with a bedroom configuration like home. If they don't have the answer right away, ask that they check and get back to you.

Think carefully before booking a room with an adjoining suite, even if it is offered as an upgrade. It may add to your stress since it creates an added opportunity for your person to wander out of the room without your knowledge.

TIP #3: Consider a disability-accessible room

Hotels throughout the United States now provide disability-accessible rooms. Many offer wider passages within the room and may come equipped with an elevated toilet seat and walk-in showers with grab bars for added safety. Some hotels may even provide temperature-control faucets and emergency call buttons in the bathroom. And, as suggested in Tip #1, remember to factor in room configuration to make sure it will match your person's needs.

TIP #4: Arrange for a room away from commotion

Getting a good night's sleep is essential for successful travel. By taking extra steps to ensure peace and quiet, you'll increase the chances that you and your person with dementia will get the rest you need.

Keep in mind that when you're in an unfamiliar location, your person may misinterpret unfamiliar sounds and images. When booking your room, speak to hotel staff and ask that you be placed in a room as far away as possible from elevators, ice machines, or other loud areas outside the building (street noise) or inside it (bar, convention, or party noise).

As night approaches, be sure to close the drapes to avoid shadows or images that may be interpreted as a stranger in the room.

TIP #5: Think about room service options

When you arrive after a long day of travel, going out to dinner can add to the growing fatigue. Room service is one way to rest and still get in a good meal.

However, if room service is not available, ask the staff if there are any local restaurants that deliver. Or, if you're traveling in the U.S., consider using a phone app for a meal delivery service. Common apps include GrubHub; DoorDash® and UberEats, just to name a few.

TIP #6: Consider a room with a coffee maker, refrigerator, microwave

Coffee makers are very common in most lodging situations. However, if you and your person have specific foods or beverages you want to have available during your stay, then a refrigerator and/or microwave is a must. Think ahead and ask about these added options.

TIP #7: Think safety

After a full day of travel, visiting people and places, you and your person are now probably exhausted. You might expect that your person is tired and will sleep soundly through the night. Yet, for some, sleep will not come easily, or they may awaken with confusion and try to leave the room.

Consider these added safety tips while in the room with your person:

- If there are two beds in the room, you should sleep in the bed closest to the door.

- Lock the door to the room and place a chair in front of the door, if you can.

- Create a set of chimes or bells on a string that you can place on the door to alert you if your person tries to exit.

- Consider using a portable door alarm or childproof door-knob cover. There are several affordable and commercially available portable door alarms designed specifically for hotel doors. (Please see the Resources section at the end of this book.) **Caution:** in an emergency, some door alarms can cause a delay when first responders answer a call for help and attempt to enter the room.

- If you wake and find your person missing, **call the front desk immediately to alert them and then dial 9-1-1.** It's better to get the police involved immediately rather than attempting to search on your own.

TIP #8: Inquire about early check-in and late departures

Flexibility is the name of the game. If you have an early arrival at your destination or you need to stop earlier in the day for an overnight stay, ask for an early check-in. With added information about your situation, the hotel staff may be able to accommodate your needs without an extra charge.

Likewise, on your day of departure, perhaps your person did not go to sleep until very late at night and you know added rest will make the day better. Call the front desk staff and request a late checkout. Even if extra fees are added, it can be well worth it if it results in successful travel.

TIP #9: Be on the lookout for service-savvy staff

Customer service is a primary focus in the hospitality industry, and the hotel business is becoming much more aware of how to better serve disabled populations.

Online reviews of hotels can help determine which accommodations will meet your needs. Sometimes a smaller, boutique hotel will provide more attentive service than a larger chain. Consider looking at reviews on websites such as TripAdvisor or Yelp! before you book a room.

TIP #10: If appropriate, let the staff know about your person's condition

Dementia is touching many people throughout the world. It is very likely that hotel staffers know a family member or friend living with dementia. If it seems necessary to share your person's diagnosis, do so in a dignified way and let the staff member know how they can be helpful. Consider using the Travel Companion Card (*Please see Chapter 1, Sample 1*) as a way to increase their awareness and understanding.

CHAPTER 14

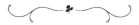

10 Tips for Dining Out

Eating out is part of almost every trip. But unfamiliar, loud, and busy restaurants can make for stressful dining for anyone. As dementia progresses, your person may also find ordering from the menu more difficult; some even forget their favorite or familiar foods. Caregivers often report that their person will try to avoid revealing their struggle by saying, "I'll have what he is having," or, "I will have the special of the day." Planning ahead for dining out will help you and your person have a better experience.

Family Favorites

Martin and Phoebe had a long tradition of taking their three adult children and families out to dinner at least monthly. Their favorite restaurant always provided them with a table for 12 in the back of the restaurant.

Yet, over the past year, Martin noticed that Phoebe – who was living with dementia – was not joining in the conversations over dinner and barely touched her meal during these gatherings. The couple's adult children were growing frustrated with Phoebe's lack of engagement during these meals and were becoming more critical of her.

Fortunately, Martin learned about the importance of planning and conducting activities during Phoebe's best time of day. He realized he could avoid overwhelming her by changing this long-standing family ritual.

He clearly communicated with his adult children about the changes that were occurring with their mom. He also let them know that he and Phoebe wanted to continue dining out with them, but now, it needed to be with only one family at a time. Martin also let the kids know that he and Phoebe preferred to meet for an early lunch rather than a Friday night dinner.

With these changes and the adult children's growing understanding of their mom's needs, this family's meal-time tradition continued for another year. More importantly, it was less stressful for Martin and more enjoyable for Phoebe.

TIP #1: Plan to eat out at the person's best time of day

We have discussed how important it is to enjoy activities, outings, and social gatherings during your person's best time of day. This is especially true of eating out. When you're planning to eat out, consider having those meals at about the time you would ordinarily eat at home.

Use caution when going out to a restaurant during high-volume lunch or dinner hours. Plan to call the restaurant directly and ask to book a reservation so that when you arrive, you can minimize or eliminate wait time.

TIP #2: Ask to be seated in a quiet place

If you call ahead for a reservation, request to be seated in a quiet area of the restaurant. Ask for a booth, if they have one – it can shield your person from additional distractions.

If you seat yourself, look for tables that are away from major traffic areas including the bar and the kitchen. If you are at a fast food restaurant, avoid a table near loud children.

TIP #3: Smaller dining groups will be best

Too many people, conversations, and noise make it almost impossible for the person living with dementia to stay focused, join in with the group, or eat their meal.

In addition, I think we can all agree that large groups at a restaurant can make it very difficult to visit with family or friends. So, before you go, consider the size of the group. If there are 10 of you, ask for one table set for four, with another nearby that's set for six.

It will be easier for your person to engage with three other people rather than with nine!

Once again, you will probably need to explain this to family and friends ahead of time.

TIP #4: When out with a group, ask someone to be your person's dining and conversation companion

When you live with dementia and find yourself in a group setting, it is often difficult to keep pace with conversations – especially when multiple conversations are happening at the same time.

Plus, as the full-time caregiver, it is also important for you to enjoy the company of friends and family. Consider asking someone else, besides you, to be your person's dining companion. Advise them that as the dinner companion, their job includes making sure your person is involved in table conversations; engaging them in one-on-one discussions and small talk; and, if needed, helping them order their meal.

Give the dining companion some of the tips you've learned about how to engage your person in conversation. You might want to consider asking a teen grandchild to be the dining companion – it may create a special connection and wonderful memories for them both.

TIP #5: Select restaurants that have pictures of food on the menu

As your person's ability to read or comprehend begins to change, you may want to look for familiar chain restaurants with menus that include pictures of the food. This allows for greater independence when ordering the meal. Sometimes, pointing to food being served at another table is another way to help your person make a selection.

TIP #6: Review the menu before you go out

Most restaurants have menus posted to their websites. Take a look before your visit. It can be very helpful to discuss choices ahead of time with your person, especially if you are not familiar with their favorite foods. Show pictures of certain foods, especially if that helps your person to remember their preferences. Gently work with your person to come up with at least a couple of options.

When you arrive at the restaurant for your meal, you can prompt your person by saying, "I am so glad we looked at the menu before we came. They have so many good things! I think you said a cheeseburger sounds good. Or do you think you might have a grilled cheese sandwich?"

TIP #7: Give choices whenever you can

If time is short and you haven't taken an advance look at the menu, try suggesting a few options as you and your person go over the menu.

For example, you might say, "I see they have a couple of your favorite dishes here. They have spaghetti with meatballs and fish and chips. What sounds good to you?" Or you can ask the wait staff, "What do you think are the two best dishes on the menu?"

After you ask your person to make a selection, *give them time to respond*. If you think they have ordered something they will not like, order something for you that you know they will eat, then plan to switch the dishes if you need to. Note that food tastes and preferences change over time. Many people living with dementia forget what they didn't like about a certain dish and now it sounds good and they eat it.

TIP #8: Avoid more than 1 glass of wine or beer, or 1 ounce of hard liquor

Enjoying a cocktail with a meal is common for many people. However, for a person with dementia, consuming more than one six-ounce glass of wine, a 12-ounce beer, or one-ounce of hard liquor may create added confusion. Watch your person closely for the effects of the alcohol.

Some ideas to keep the adult beverages to a minimum include:

- Ordering your cocktail with the meal

- Asking the wait staff or bartender for a list of 'mocktails'

- Inquiring if the bar or restaurant serves non-alcoholic beer or wine

- Asking if hard liquor can be watered-down in the next drink, or

- Selecting restaurants that do not serve liquor.

It's important to plan ahead, so you're not in the position of having to police your person's alcohol consumption.

TIP #9: Utilize the travel companion card if your person becomes undignified

It may be helpful from the start to let your servers know how much you appreciate their patience and understanding during the dining experience. If your person becomes impatient while waiting for food, or is critical of the wait staff, handing them your Travel Companion Card may do the trick to raise awareness and defuse the situation. As you present the card, you might add, "I'm sorry, this is just a bad day (or a bad time). I appreciate all you are doing."

TIP #10: Think ahead of how to manage the bill when the person with dementia insists on paying

For many, it is fairly customary for a man to pay for the meal. Yet, when the man has dementia, there can be some added confusion when it comes time to settle the bill. With his dignity in mind, let him pay, while offering your assistance in calculating the tip. If he resists, have cash handy and either discreetly leave it on the table, or as you get to the car, excuse yourself by saying you left something behind. Go back into the restaurant and pay for the meal. Leave a good tip – it's a great way to show your gratitude to the staff who go the extra mile to make your dining experience pleasurable.

Another idea: slip the wait staff your credit card ahead of time. Then excuse yourself to use the restroom, find your waiter or waitress, and ask them to charge it to your card. If your person asks about the bill, you can say, "The meal has already been taken care of! Aren't we lucky?"

CHAPTER 15

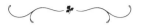

10 Tips for Hiring a Travel Companion

Whether you're on a flight from one city to the next or an extended road trip, a travel companion can make all the difference in reducing the stress of travel. No matter if it's a family member, a friend, or a professional travel companion, you will want to do your homework and carefully decide who can best provide the support you need.

TIP #1: Create a job description for the travel companion

This may sound ridiculous, but it's important to think about specifics and delve deeply into what you and your person need to make this trip successful.

For a single person with mild cognitive impairment, a travel companion might be someone who:

- Is willing to join in a fun experience with you

- Has enough travel savvy to negotiate and problem-solve for unexpected delays or changes in plans

- Can manage the details of the itinerary

- Can assist with reminders for wake-up, excursions, taking medications, and more.

For the person with moderate dementia, the travel companion's role may include:

- Keeping your person company and meaningfully occupied when the caregiver steps away or goes out alone

- Assisting your person with dressing and grooming tasks

- Assisting with toileting or bathing, or

- Administering medication.

For someone with advanced dementia, the travel companion might need to be a licensed nurse who can assist with giving medication, assist with meals and eating, or changing a brief.

Take your time and think through what you need and, more importantly, what you **expect** a travel companion to do to assist you. The tasks you identify will help you decide if the travel companion could be a friend or family member, or should have a nursing license, a caregiver certificate, CPR training, or other certifications. This will help you get the right person with the right skills and a better result all around.

TIP #2: Think about the kind of travel companion your person will like and accept

Many family caregivers are quick to say, "My [mom, dad, spouse] will NEVER accept help!"

However, you – as an informed caregiver – have probably found ways to help your person live well and accept help, even if it's in an indirect way.

Here are some additional ideas to consider as you think about what your person may need or will accept:

- You have mild cognitive impairment and want to take that bucket-list trip 'down under' to Australia. You know it will be demanding. Your best friend loves to travel but does not have the funds to pay for the trip. Could you ask him to join you and assist as needed, in exchange for paying for the trip?

- You think your wife is too modest to let someone assist her in the shower, but you know she loves to visit with people. As you think about the kind of companion you want for her, remember that strong social skills on the part of the travel companion will be a must. If you want the companion to help her with bathing or grooming, you may want to take an extra step and make sure the candidate you're considering is a certified nursing assistant or licensed caregiver.

- Your mother loves her youngest college-age granddaughter, Katie. You notice how your mom easily goes along with whatever Katie suggests. Think about asking Katie if she might join as the travel companion and schedule the trip over one of Katie's college breaks.

- Your husband was once an executive; introducing the travel companion as a personal assistant or concierge may be a way to preserve his dignity and provide the help he needs. In this case, be sure to look for a 'polished' travel companion.

- Your dad seems to gravitate toward younger people, particularly women because he says they are "fun!" Can you find a younger travel companion who likes to engage with your dad and create fun in a safe and meaningful way?

TIP #3: Begin the search for a travel companion

If you have identified a family member or a friend as a potential companion, ask them, in a kind and forthright way, if they truly are up for the task. Don't expect them to do this for free. Yes, you hope that this individual will have fun and will enjoy the trip, but your primary purpose for bringing them along is to help you and your person.

In addition to covering the companion's travel expenses, ask what they think would be a fair wage. Make sure they understand this is a job, not an expense-free vacation with no responsibilities.

Perhaps you intend to seek the assistance of a home care company or a travel company to find a companion. **You must still do your homework**. Be sure the person you hire has the skills you need. **This is not the time to make a decision solely on price.** You need both the quality and know-how for the tasks you have identified – especially if your person needs hand-on personal or medical care. Expect to pay more for that kind of attention. Keep in mind, this is a trip you have decided to take; see it as an investment and get the best help you can find.

TIP #4: Don't be afraid to interview multiple agencies to compare

Interview multiple non-medical home care companies using a questionnaire that allows you to compare one service with another. For example, you will want to know:

- How they provide background checks on their employees

- What kind of certification(s) does the candidate possess

- How many trips the candidate has completed as a travel companion

- The company's safety record for its travel companions

- The type of insurance the company carries, and

- The company's policy for a companion who abruptly leaves an assignment.

No matter which non-medical home care company you choose, plan to carefully interview each and every candidate. In addition to the companion's travel and/or technical skills, you need to **drill them about what they know about dementia**. Get a sense of how flexible they are. If they have limited to no experience in caring for or traveling with a person with dementia, a long trip is not the time for an experimental engagement.

Perhaps you can create some scenarios that reflect what you experience on a daily basis. Use these during the interview to see how the candidate companion would respond to these situations.

Note: *finding a male companion may take a bit more time since there is often a limited supply of men who do this work.*

TIP #5: Try out the travel companion before the trip

Just as you may have tried a staycation before embarking on a big trip, you may want to have the travel companion spend some time with your person before you leave. Since you are traveling as a unit, schedule a visit of two-to-four hours, and plan to be present most of the time. Not only do you need to like and get along with this individual, but your person needs to feel comfortable, as well.

Before the visit, prepare the travel companion by providing information about you and especially your person. Let them know a bit about who your loved one is. Write out a brief life story to assist the companion in understanding more about your person, such as where they grew up; favorite childhood memories; work history; family members they like to talk about; other favorite people; favorite stories; and favorite music, TV, movies, sports, activities, etc. Watch carefully for how the companion interacts with your person. You may find it helpful to schedule several visits well before the trip, allowing your person to be more familiar and comfortable when travel begins.

Note: there are numerous life story formats available for free online.

TIP #6: Consider if you will you require the companion to be travel savvy

If you are a novice or nervous traveler, you may want added travel skills and finesse from your hired companion, over and above what's covered in the job description you prepared.

Be sure to let the companion know what you will require of them during travel. For example, will you expect the companion to be in charge of the luggage? Do you want them to handle check-in at airports, hotels, and excursions? Will they be managing travel documents, making reservations or assisting in making changes when travel is delayed or canceled?

The clearer you are about your expectations; the better chance the companion has to provide the level of service you're looking for.

TIP #7: Be sure the companion has a sense of your person's daily routine and preferences

In addition to providing your person's life story, it is essential for the travel companion to know your person's usual routine and how to best support it.

Think about writing out the daily routine you use at home. The travel companion (family member, friend or professional) can use this as a guide during travel. Include things as simple as, "John likes an ice cube in his black coffee in the morning." "Mary likes to take her pills with a bowl of vanilla ice cream." "Please lay out her clothing in the order that she puts it on." "Bill likes to shower after he eats breakfast in the morning."

TIP #8: Find out if the travel companion is prepared to keep your person occupied

Do not assume the travel companion knows how to meaningfully engage with your person. (This is yet another reason to have the person visit a few times before the trip). While watching a bit of TV is okay, if that is the only thing they do during the trip, this is expensive respite care!

Just as you've shared the personal side through the life story, you can also provide the companion with the list of favorite activities you've already compiled (please see Chapter 9's Tips for Keeping Your Person Occupied During Travel).

For example, perhaps your husband once liked to golf. During a day at sea, the travel companion knows she can invite him to go to the upper deck to check out the driving range and putting green. Off they go, while you enjoy some time at the spa or by the pool with a book. Later, when you notice your husband is too tired to join the family for dinner, the companion is primed to say, "Let's order a pizza and watch that great John Wayne movie" on the tablet contained in your travel activities bag.

Just as you have prepared the travel activities and props, make sure your travel companion has access to these things and knows how and when to introduce them.

TIP #9: Ensure the companion knows how to intervene if your person gets upset

People living with dementia have more difficulty coping with stress. As you've learned, sources of stress are varied and may include fatigue, change in the environment, becoming overwhelmed with a task, or having difficulty understanding a particular situation.

There can also be physical causes that lead to upset. These might include pain, constipation, or even hunger. Since the person has more difficulty managing these sources of stress or unmet physical needs and cannot fully communicate the upset, you are more likely to see unwanted behaviors that are uncharacteristic for the person. Whether it is confusion or inability to fully express their needs, "behavioral expressions" become the way the person will respond. Do not think of these expressions as willful behaviors; rather, help your companion interpret them as a form of communication in a person with a serious brain illness.

Share with the companion the effective techniques you've learned or created that help keep your person comfortable and/or distracted when the upset occurs.

TIP #10: Let the companion know the 'triggers' to be aware of and avoid

Some people living with dementia will have situations, topics, or chronic health conditions that trigger upset if not managed well. In particular, untreated pain can lead to irritability or refusal to participate in activities. The time of day can also be a trigger for upset since it can represent fatigue and the need for rest or a nap. For some, asking too many questions can create upset.

For those with hallucinations, determine if what the person sees is upsetting to them. For someone with Lewy Body Dementia who frequently sees imaginary cats running about, it would be important to ask her if the cats are bothering her. If they are, you might respond by saying, "I opened the door so they would leave and not annoy you anymore." Ask the companion to be just as creative and respectful in responding to your person. Remind the companion that telling your person there are no cats will not be helpful.

Likewise, if the person has delusions – fixed false beliefs – take time to determine how upsetting these are and let the travel companion know. For example, a woman with vascular dementia might become upset when she tries to call her parents. Rather than explaining that they have been deceased for years, her daughter calmly responds, "I bet they are out running errands. You know what busy people they are." If it's a technique that works, make sure the travel companion knows about it and can use it.

As dementia progresses, normal responses in communication frequently do not work. An effective strategy is to enter into your person's reality with 'therapeutic fibbing.' It takes practice but tends to reduce conflict. Some of you may find it uncomfortable to consider answering your person with un-truths. Remember, that for both you and the travel companion, the goal is about keeping the person comfortable. Trying to get your person to join your reality will result in frustration and upset for everyone.

Bottom line: if you know what commonly triggers behavioral expressions in your person, let your travel companion (and family members) know so they can use these same strategies to keep your person comfortable.

CHAPTER 16

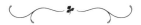

10 Tips for Finding Respite Care Options

Not everyone living with dementia will be able to travel. But you, as the caregiver, may need to travel for a variety of reasons: personal desires; a break from the demands of caregiving; or milestone celebrations with family and friends. If you need a break, give yourself permission to take one. Overcome the guilt. You are in a tough situation and you need to have a life beyond your role as a caregiver. Ask yourself, "If my person (parent, spouse, sibling) was still able to see the situation for what it is now, and knew I wanted to take this trip, what would they tell me?" There's a good chance the answer would be, "Yes, please take the trip." Remember, your person did not want to have dementia and probably did not want you to sacrifice your hopes and dreams, either. ***It is okay to travel without your person.***

Be prepared for the likelihood that family and friends might not understand why your person can no longer travel. Ongoing and honest communication will aid in helping them to understand and support your decision.

To make your own travel plans a reality ***now*** is the time to find the respite care that will be best for your person. And since emergency travel situations can happen, it is wise to pre-select options in advance should the need arise. This process can be quite involved and takes time.

Use these 10 tips to help you with your planning.

Traveling Without Him

Janelle and Tony have been married for 20 years. Tony, a retired salesman, was diagnosed with early-stage Alzheimer's disease in the past year. Janelle works from home about 32 hours a week. Recently, her company asked her to travel to a five-day training conference in New York City. Janelle not only wanted to attend the conference to advance her knowledge but quite honestly, she was also looking for a break as well.

Janelle knew that Tony could not stay alone, and they had a very limited network of friends they could ask for help. She contacted Tony's two adult children to ask if he could either travel to them and stay for the week, or if they could take time off to come and stay with their dad. Neither child was able to help. While she was disappointed, Janelle decided to put her efforts into finding the right respite care for her husband.

Janelle began to consider options for either in-home care or respite care in a residential community and sought input from others in her support group. One group member shared her recent, positive experience with a residential community for her husband. As Janelle made calls, interviewed home care companies and visited residential communities, she quickly realized that since Tony was such a social and active guy, that the residential option would be best for him.

Janelle prepared Tony for the adventure they were both going to have in the next few days. She had him select his clothing and helped him to pack for his weeklong lodging. She made sure the staff knew a bit more about her husband, particularly the food he loved, along with his favorite activities and topics to discuss. Each night, Janelle called her husband to share her day while reminding him she would be home soon. The staff at the residential setting sent a daily photo to Janelle's cell phone showing Tony engaged with other residents.

The week passed quickly. Janelle returned to Tony, who successfully made it through the week and created some new friends. Janelle now knows she will probably be able to use respite care in the future. She also is aware of how much better she feels having had a weeklong break from her caregiving role.

TIP #1: Outline the type of help your person needs while you are gone

Early in dementia, companionship, transportation, and help with household chores may be all you need. By the time the disease reaches a moderate stage, your person probably needs either reminders or help with grooming, dressing, bathing and may even need reminders to eat. In the advanced stage, your person will need help with the full range of everyday tasks and will likely get the best care in a residential setting with skilled caregivers. (*Please see Chapter 1, Table 1, Stages of Dementia.*)

Make a list of the chores or tasks your person must have help with. Home care agencies and residential communities will ask this question – the list you create will help you think clearly as you begin to research your options.

TIP #2: Determine if a family member or friend can help out

Some families and friends, who are well-informed and supportive of the primary caregiver, may offer to stay with your person even before you ask. If they don't offer right away, don't be afraid to ask. Be honest about what you need from them and for how long. Be clear about other duties may be necessary, from household chores and cooking meals to assistance with personal care.

Here are a few examples:

- The person living with dementia attends an Adult Day Care program five-days a week from 9:00 a.m. to 3:00 p.m. You need your sister to stay with your mom, get your mom ready to go by 8:30 a.m., drop her off at Day Care, and pick her up by 3:00 p.m. Your sister will also need to stay with your mom for the rest of the day, night, and weekend. Can she adjust her work hours for a week?

- Your spouse needs 24/7 supervision and companionship. You ask your son to stay for the entire week, but you also let him know you have scheduled your husband's usual home care companion to come in to give your son a break on Monday, Wednesday, and Friday from 10:00 a.m. to 2:00 p.m. The companion will help your dad to take a shower during the visits.

With this kind of support already in place, would your son be willing to fly out for a week to stay?

- You are going out-of-town to celebrate your grandson's graduation from medical school. Your wife has moderate dementia but loves spending time with her sister, who lives in town. You ask your sister-in-law if she would be willing to invite your wife to stay in her home for five days while you travel to the graduation in Miami. You let your sister-in-law know that your wife needs reminders to bathe and change into her nightgown at night. The sister will also need to give your wife her daily medications, which you have thoughtfully arranged in a pillbox. You also share your wife's daily routine that includes the shows she likes to watch on TV. With these accommodations in mind, can your sister-in-law take your wife for five days?

TIP #3: Use a full-time or supplemental companion from an agency or Adult Day Health Care

Most family members or friends who offer to provide respite care are not prepared for the 24/7 demands that you have come to understand. It can be very helpful to supplement their respite care by bringing in a companion or bath aid from a home care agency during your time away.

It is best to introduce home care prior to your planned respite, so your person has a chance to become familiar with the paid companion. Many non-medical home care companies have a two-day per week, four-hour minimum requirement.

Perhaps a working adult child cannot take time off from work but is willing to stay with your person. You might consider hiring a paid companion who can come in during your adult child's working hours. That may be enough to keep your loved one at home, with your adult child overseeing care for the rest of the time.

Another option in many areas is an Adult Day Health Care program. These programs generally operate Monday through Friday, from 7:00 a.m. to 6:00 p.m. In addition to many group activities and engagement opportunities available through these programs, a registered nurse is onsite to give medications and meals are provided. Some programs offer transportation services and may assist with showers, as well. If you plan to use Adult Day Health Care to supplement the respite period, enroll your person well ahead of your planned respite so they have time to adjust to this setting.

TIP #4: Do your homework and interview at least two or three non-medical home care agencies

Some caregivers may decide to use a live-in companion during the respite period because they know their loved one is more comfortable in the home setting. Just as you have identified your person's needs for family and friends, you should provide this list as you interview home care agencies. For those who require hands-on care such as bathing, incontinence care, assistance with getting out of a chair or walking, a certified nursing assistant (CNA) will be best.

Plan to interview a few home care agencies. You're looking not only for pricing and availability; most importantly, you need to assess their staff's ability to meet the needs of your person.

Just as you would when hiring a travel companion, you will want to know how the agency provides background checks and how it trains staff in dementia care. Ask about the agency's ability to replace a paid companion if your person does not get along with the one assigned. Determine if the agency can cover any needs that arise during the night and how they will stay in touch with you in case of an emergency.

TIP #5: If at-home care doesn't work, consider a residential setting

Sometimes staying at home is **not** the best option. Residential centers and homes may provide a more supportive and engaging setting. Give focused thought to whether you need a community that provides a memory care option. Generally, staff in memory care programs have added education and are better equipped to care for the person with moderate to advanced dementia.

Research your options carefully. Many caregivers will check with their support group or other caregivers who have used these options. You can also contact your local Alzheimer's Association (www.alz.org) or Area Agency on Aging (www.n4a.org) to find options in their area. (Please see Resources: General Caregiver Services and Respite Care.)

TIP #6: Call before looking at residential care options

Before you start to visit residential options, make calls to see if respite care is even available. For many residential settings, respite care is conditional, based upon bed or room availability. Make sure the setting can provide the type of care your person needs.

TIP #7: Be sure to visit several places

By visiting various settings, you will get a better sense of whether you will be comfortable leaving your person for a week or two. During your visit, keep these pointers in mind:

- Look beyond the décor.

- Watch carefully how staff engage other residents.

- Meet with activities staff and ask what types of activities are offered.

- Eat a meal with residents to see if the food is decent and mealtime is pleasant.

- Ask staffers if they like their jobs (and notice if they smile while they are working).

- Inquire about how long the administrator has been there.

- Ask how staff are educated about dementia and how they get to know their residents.

Resist the temptation to tell yourself, "My person will never be happy here," or "My person is not as bad off as the rest of these people." People living with dementia are resilient. In fact, most of them adapt nicely to these settings, making them an acceptable choice for residential respite care.

Some family caregivers have found that, upon their return from a trip, their loved one has settled into this new setting nicely. This could be a turning point for the caregiver, inviting a new willingness to consider long term placement. For others, it is simply a good reminder that their person can adapt to a new setting and be comfortable.

TIP #8: Think twice before taking your person along to visit respite providers

Unless your person is early in their dementia and agrees to a stay in a residential setting while you go away, bringing your person along as you check out options is generally not a good idea. If your person truly needs this level of supervisory care and support, they are usually beyond the ability to determine what setting is right for them.

If you try to explain that your person will stay there while you go away, your person is likely to shoot down the whole idea immediately. You're then facing your last resort: trying to reason, convince or coerce your person. This will not work and now, you may have an unwanted argument on your hands.

Once you have decided on the location, try taking your person for lunch at the community. Before you do, though, please carefully evaluate whether this is a good move. If your person complains about the lunchtime visit or food, you may find yourself having to eliminate what might have been a good option.

TIP #9: Provide a detailed schedule of your person's routines, likes/dislikes, and food preferences

Your person's success during this respite stay also depends on how quickly the staff can learn about your person and support your person's routine. Once again, a completed Life Story that spells out your person's favorites, preferences, and aversions will aid in helping your person connect with the paid companion, residential staff, and even family members.

Routine, combined with meaningful engagement, will make your person more comfortable during your absence.

TIP #10: Don't pre-announce the respite plans too far in advance

People living with dementia lose their ability to understand time relationships. Even tracking the difference between two weeks versus two days can be confusing.

If you announce the plans too soon, be prepared to hear the repeated questions like...

- "Where are you going?"

- "When are you going?"

- "When is Bonnie coming to visit?"

- "I am NOT going to that home you found!"

For some, you may need to wait until the day of the trip to announce the plan. Or perhaps you'll decide that you do not need to announce the plan at all. Think about this carefully. There's no reason to add unnecessary anxiety for either of you.

CHAPTER 17

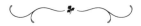

10 Tips for Using a Travel Agent

We live in an era in which so much travel information is at our fingertips via the web. Yet, travel agents are still able to play a powerful role in planning travel for people living with dementia. They can make suggestions and arrangements for accommodations that might not have occurred to you. They can also help you save time and money, address your specific needs, and solve problems – especially in the face of canceled or delayed travel. A travel agent can often readily rebook most reservations, allowing you, the caregiver, to stay focused on the person living with dementia.

These tips will help you get the most out of your travel agent:

TIP #1: Select a travel agent who specializes in the type of travel you want

Many people find a travel agent through the suggestion of a family member or friend. Others may take advantage of membership in programs such as AAA or American Express.

There is a growing number of travel agents who specialize in services for those with disabilities, although the focus tends to be on physical disability rather than cognitive disability. (Don't rule out the physical-disability travel agents – they can provide great assistance whether your person needs basic medical equipment like wheelchair transport, or more advanced needs like oxygen, hospital beds, or lifts.)

Think about the type of travel you are looking for and match that to the agent who is most knowledgeable. For example, a couple thinking about taking a cruise will probably do better on a smaller ship than a larger one that draws families. Look for agents who focus solely on cruising or small group travel.

If you are traveling with young family members, an agent with experience may suggest a cruise line or ship that can meet the needs of both the younger and older passengers, knowing that the grandmother with dementia will need access to quieter spaces through the day and a quiet dinner in the evening.

There is at least one dementia specialty travel agent now offering cruises for people living with dementia, family caregivers and other frail elders. Registered Nurse Kathy Shoaf owns Elite Cruises and Vacations and hosts numerous dementia-capable cruises throughout the year (http://www.elitecruisesandvacationstravel.com/).

Many people will elect not to use a travel agent if only booking a flight or hotel room. In these situations, rather than working solely online, it is best to call the company directly and speak with a customer service representative. These representatives can generally assist with additional accommodations you have determined will be needed. But keep in mind that a good travel agent may have access to many more resources than what you might find on a website. While there may be a fee for their services, it will be worth it to get the right hotel in the perfect location or flight with the best times or connections. **Bonus:** for foreign travel, an agent will also help you with advice on health advisories, vaccinations, added health insurance, passports or visa applications.

TIP #2: Let the travel agent reduce your stress!

As a family caregiver, time is certainly precious. A travel agent can be helpful when learning about your travel needs and can research the best options for you. In addition to saving time, travel agents know how to work with various budgets. They may have access to better pricing or can extend corporate rates for hotels, car rentals, free parking, and more. Based on your stated needs, they may recommend upgrades which, while more expensive, may add to your person's comfort.

TIP #3: Communicate honestly with your agent about the needs of your person

It is important, when working with a travel agent, that you are upfront about the needs of you and your person. Don't expect that they will understand how dementia is impacting you, let alone your person.

To help them do a good job for you, it is essential you provide the following information to the agent:

- Diagnosis of Alzheimer's disease/dementia and any special needs your person may have

- Best time of the day for travel and excursions

- Length of time your person can tolerate travel or excursions

- Routines that will make travel better

- Preference for hotel room/cruise cabin layout (*Please see Chapter 12, 10 Tips for Hotel Stays*)

- Added services you will need in airports, train terminals, cruise ships, etc. Ask about wheelchair assistance for security, check-in, and arrivals. Programs that provide expedited wait times will minimize added fatigue and frustration.

- Any special medical equipment e.g. hospital bed, wheelchair, walker, scooter, elevated toilet seat, oxygen, etc.

- Information about other travel companions or family joining in the trip.

TIP #4: Let the agent notify vendors about your special needs

Most employees in the travel industry want to provide a high level of customer service. While they may not be as knowledgeable about dementia as you are, they can give added notice to airlines, cruise lines, and other travel vendors (e.g. hotels, tour operators, etc.). Those 'travel notes' will remind everyone to slow down, be patient and respectful, and keep a more watchful eye on the person.

Keep in mind that sometimes these requests may not be seen by the airline, cruise line, or hotel. For an added measure of confidence in your plans, be sure to check with vendors to make sure the travel notes have been received.

TIP #5: Use the agent's wealth of experience to find the most efficient and effective means of travel

As mentioned, providing the travel agent with your person's best time of day for travel and how much activity they can tolerate each day during travel will allow the agent to create a plan that is more finely tuned to your person. Examples may include:

- A long-haul trip that is divided into two days to allow for a sleepover in a hotel airport.

- A private excursion of 90-minutes in length, rather than the usual four to six-hour excursion.

- Private ground transport scheduled at all stops during the trip.

- Luggage shipped in advance, to limit additional time spent claiming bags.

- A three-day road trip mapped out in advance, with five hours of drive time each day and a comfortable hotel room booked near good dining options.

- Dining options and alternatives that suit your person's usual schedule.

TIP #6: Let the agent connect you to concierge services

As mentioned in Tip #2, services that reduce your stress may be a good investment. A travel concierge may be able to handle changes in itinerary, locate laundry services, book transportation, and deal with other issues that may arise while you and your person are traveling.

Once again, the focus is not on cost but accommodating the needs of the person living with dementia. The more flexible the travel, the better for all.

TIP #7: Let the agent explore the value of upgrades and value-add travel

Most of us are used to shopping for travel based on price and availability. But as we have discussed, for people living with dementia, the top considerations should be comfort and convenience.

Take a moment to review Chapter 4, *Five Tips to Manage Added Stressors Created by Travel*. You might want to share some or all of that information with your travel agent, so they can assist you in evaluating paid upgrades and determining if you can factor them into your travel budget.

Upgrades to consider include:

- Premium economy seats or business class on airlines for more legroom and wider seats

- Faster check-in/check-out

- Fast-track security (TSA in the United States)

- Faster immigration checks (Global Entry, part of U.S. Customs and Border Patrol, https://www.cbp.gov/travel/trusted-traveler-programs/global-entry)

- Club facilities in the airport or train station lounge areas

- Priority baggage assistance

- Luxury car transport

- Early check-in/late check-out

- An upgraded hotel that is more comfortable and includes breakfast.

TIP #8: Let the agent help you invest in the best travel insurance

Many people never consider purchasing travel insurance. But those living with dementia and other pre-existing medical conditions will find this option to be very beneficial – especially for planned (and expensive) trips.

Ask your travel agent about the best options to cover trip cancellation, emergency medical coverage and/or medical evacuation. This additional insurance will provide you peace of mind should something unforeseen arise before or during your travels.

Note: Medicare, Medicare Supplements (Part B) and Commercial insurance ***may have limited to no coverage depending on where you are traveling***. It is important to contact your medical insurance carrier prior to travel to determine what medical care, if any, is covered during domestic travel. You can also visit www.medicare.gov/coverage/travel for more information.

Remember that travel insurance and medical insurance are very different products. Clarify your needs with your travel agent.

TIP #9: Book private tours that accommodate your needs

Whether traveling separately or with a group, booking private tours can help minimize added stress caused by large groups and long tours that create too much demand. Travel agents are knowledgeable about how to connect you to private tour operators who can meet you at your destination and tailor your excursion, even as the time unfolds.

They will provide specific times that are best for pick up; inform you of group size; tell you about the length of the outing; allow plenty of time to return to your hotel or ship; and more. While this service may cost more, you and your loved one will probably feel far more at ease.

TIP #10: Get assistance in organizing your documents

Depending on the length of your trip and the number of vendors involved, having the added assistance of printing and organizing your documents will be most helpful. While electronic tickets and documents are becoming the norm, having printed documents may still be your best option. As you work with your travel agent, let them know that you would appreciate detailed, printed travel documents. (*Please see Chapter 8, 10 Essential Documents to Carry When You Travel.*)

CHAPTER 18

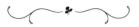

10 Tips for Booking Air Travel

Air travel is one of the most common ways that people transit the world. However, with overcrowded planes and airports, it is essential to do your homework before you book your trip.

TIP #1: Make an honest appraisal to determine if your person can fly alone (_Please see Table 2, in Chapter 2, Travel Support for Dementia_**).**

If you decide to let your loved one travel alone, you should, _**at a minimum**_, plan to accompany them to the departure gate and stay there until the plane has left the gate. On the arrival side, be sure to have a family member or friend meet your person **at the gate**. On either end of the trip, you will need a gate pass from the designated airline to be allowed access to the secure gate areas. You should also take a picture of your person the day of the flight in the clothes they wear should you need to notify security.

Keep in mind that on occasion, the plane may have to make an unexpected diversion. While this is rare, ask yourself if your person could ask effectively for assistance. _**If the short answer is "NO," then your loved one should not fly alone.**_

You can also use a flight tracker app to track the flight for unexpected delays, diversions, etc.

TIP #2: If booking a ticket online, be sure to look for "special assistance" to note your person's condition

This is critical – it notifies the gate and flight crew that added assistance may be needed. There is no airline industry standard that defines how to identify or record cognitive impairment in a passenger. Each airline will use different terminology, making it challenging to find and ask for added assistance.

When you search the airline website, take a look for special assistance by looking for words such as "accessible travel," "special service," "special needs travel," or "senior travel." Note that airlines make much more information available about physical needs and support versus cognitive needs. And, if "cognitive impairment" is listed, it is likely to either be non-specific or will lump together a range of individual needs including autism, intellectual and developmental disability, and dementia.

Yet, it is imperative the airline know, ahead of time, of any unique needs your person may have – ***especially if you are planning to send the person on the flight alone*** (although you've read by now to think twice about this!).

TIP #3: Consider calling the airline directly or working with your travel agent to book flights

Quite honestly, this might be the easiest way to ensure the airline will do the extra work involved in noting your person's special needs. It matters because some airlines provide additional support on their own while others have partnerships with contractors like Global Airport Concierge to provide additional services. The airline or your travel agent will be more familiar with additional services, if available or needed, and how to communicate with them.

Whenever possible, fly direct or connect in larger hubs to avoid using smaller, regional jets. Often, the smaller jets depart from a different concourse, far from connecting flights. Some will not have jet bridges, instead requiring passengers to board the plane by climbing stairs. Avoid this whenever possible.

TIP #4: Pre-arrange seats

Whether booking online or working directly with the airline or travel agent, it is best to book a seat that will optimize the comfort and convenience for you and your person. When booking online, you will be provided with the plane's configuration. Think about minimizing disruption by having your person sit by the window or in the middle, so there won't be other passengers climbing over your person when they need to stretch or use the restroom. In this situation, you will want to have adjoining seats.

Being closer to the toilet is helpful for many, so getting seats near the front of the plane is ideal. However, these are now considered premium seats and will often have an added charge. While emergency rows do provide extra space, if your person cannot follow instructions and assist with a potential evacuation, they should not be seated in those rows. You can also look at seat maps by searching www.seatguru.com.

For more information about how the airline can support the needs of those with an identified disability such as dementia, visit https://www.transportation.gov/individuals/aviation-consumer-protection/traveling-disability.

TIP #5: Consider upgrading your seats to premium economy or business class

As mentioned previously, the more comfortable you are inflight, the better the trip will be – especially during longer flights. This will also be helpful if you need to make connections along the way since you and your person will be in the group that deplanes first. Be sure to request early boarding at the time you book your flight. Remember to bring it up again at the airport when checking in or when you arrive at the gate.

TIP #6: Look for flights that depart during your person's best time of the day

For most people living with dementia, this will mean flights between the hours of 10:00 a.m. and 3:00 p.m. In general, these will be less busy times in the airports, especially when flying mid-week (Tuesday – Thursday) and on Saturday. However, as more people take to the air, even these times and days are busier than in the past. Use your best judgment but know that if you are booking early-morning flights, getting your loved one up in the middle of the night may be difficult.

TIP #7: Consider flexible schedules and stop-overs for longer or connecting flights

Some find it helpful to break up long-haul flights with stopovers to allow your person to gradually adjust to changing time zones. With connecting flights, be sure to schedule enough time to break up travel. You'll also want to avoid rushing to your next flight or having too much time on the ground between flights.

When booking long-haul flights, or connecting flights with long layovers, investigate if the airline has a club that you can utilize while you wait for your flight. If you're not already a member, many airlines will offer a paid, one-day pass to use their club. It's a valuable perk since clubs can offer a quieter location, provide refreshments and the use of comfortable restrooms (and sometimes showers) for customers.

TIP #8: Purchase insurance for the flight

Most airlines provide this as an option. Be sure to read the fine print so you know what situations apply. Do your homework and seek advice about purchasing the right type of coverage for you and your person. Once again, you may want to consult with your travel agent or call the airline directly.

TIP #9: Consider taking a short flight as a trial run

Just as you might try a staycation before the trip, you may also want to experiment with a shorter trip via air before you book a longer one. You'll want to evaluate how your person does while passing through security, waiting at the gate and during the flight. In addition, you also want to evaluate **your** stress level as well. During this trial run, you can think about how you will manage a longer flight, from the time you leave for the airport through the end of the trip.

TIP #10: Consider the need for an extra travel companion

An additional travel companion can be very helpful during long trips and/or to assist with check-in, luggage, arrival, bathroom assistance, or to keep an additional watchful eye on your person so they remain safe and comfortable. This will also allow you to feel more at ease. As discussed in Chapter 14, *10 Tips to Hiring a Travel Companion*, be very clear about what you need from this companion and be sure to communicate it well in advance.

CHAPTER 19

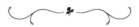

10 Tips for Navigating the Airport

Unless you are flying out of a small regional airport, most major airports are loud, overwhelming and confusing – especially to the older and/or novice traveler. As noted in Chapter 4, *5 Tips and Solutions for Managing the Added Stress Created by Travel*, the person living with dementia is more easily stressed by their environment. These tips will assist to minimize the overwhelm that can result in anxiety and upset.

TIP #1: Plan to arrive at least two hours in advance

For international travel, a minimum of three-hours is often suggested. You will be more relaxed knowing that you are not rushed for time. Remember, if you get frazzled, so will your loved one.

TIP #2: Get assistance with your luggage so you can focus on checking in

If porter service is available, use it. This will allow you (or a travel companion) to focus on checking in, getting through security and to your gate.

Don't forget that as you plan for your travel, you may want to ship your luggage ahead of time so that all you have with you is a carry-on bag. Be sure, as you check in, to remind the gate agent that you are requesting early boarding. Check to make sure that any special requests for the assistance you made ahead of time are noted in the record. If not, ask that the agent put them in the record now.

TIP #3: Ask for a skycap or wheelchair transport to move through security lines quickly

This can be tricky since the person living with dementia generally will not need the transport for mobility and might not understand you are using this service to expedite the security process. If you anticipate this to be a problem, consider purchasing a TSA Precheck (https://www.cbp.gov/travel/trusted-traveler-programs/global-entry/tsa-precheck) or Global Entry pass (https://www.cbp.gov/travel/trusted-traveler-programs/global-entry/how-apply) several months ahead of your trip. Or, YOU ask to use the wheelchair transport, even if your person simply walks alongside it. The goal is to expedite security. You don't need to explain it to your loved one; just be very matter of fact about the use of the skycap.

Be sure to remain with your person during the **_entire_** security process. Show the TSA or security staff the companion card that identifies your person as one who needs additional support and patience. Let the personnel know that you cannot be separated from your person. If your person has particular sensitivities (for example, dislikes being touched) or communication challenges (cannot follow commands), be sure security personnel is aware. Ask to move through security ahead of your person so you can keep an eye on them as they go through the screening process.

Just as you have communicated with the TSA/security team, help the skycap know how to communicate with your person. Be prepared to tip well for good service and patience.

TIP #4: Be sure you carry all travel documents and identification cards

Take your time and be sure you collect **all** your belongings before heading to the gate. For the person with dementia who insists on carrying their own documents, some families report success using a plastic pocket, attached to a lanyard and worn around the neck, to tuck away travel documents. Do not rush! Be sure to check that all documents and IDs are returned to the lanyard before leaving the security area.

TIP #5: Purchase snacks and beverages

If you did not bring snacks from home, plan to pick some up now, since food selections onboard an aircraft can be limited. Because it can take up to an hour before inflight beverage service begins, remember to also purchase favorite fluids to bring on board.

Don't let your person go to a gift shop or eatery alone and think they will make their way back to the gate. They won't. Instead, stay with your loved one at all times.

TIP #6: Use the restroom before boarding – even if you don't think you need to!

While restricting fluids is generally frowned upon, it is recommended to limit fluid on the day of travel. Even so, try to use the restroom before boarding. Family restrooms are now available in most airports, and they are particularly useful for the person who needs assistance. Remember that toileting can take added time and you don't want to rush your person.

Be sure you have packed extra incontinence products and clothing in case your person may need them during travel (please see Chapter 11, 10 Tips for Managing Continence During Travel). Do not ask a stranger to watch your person while you use the toilet. Your person will walk away and is at risk of getting lost.

Gone in an Instant

Paula and Stan set out for a fabulous trip to Hawaii despite Stan's obvious confusion. Stan had never been diagnosed with a dementia and Paula had little understanding of the condition. What was about to unfold in a few short moments underscored the fact that Paula was completely unprepared.

The couple arrived in Honolulu and waited for their connecting flight. After finishing lunch, Paula asked Stan to wait for her outside the ladies' restroom while she used the facilities. When Paula came out, Stan was nowhere to be found. She rushed to their gate thinking that she would find Stan. She began asking other passengers if they had seen her husband. Finally, she called security who launched a search for Stan. Some two hours later, Stan was found – in Maui!

Paula did not understand Stan's profound memory loss or his ability to follow instructions. Stan did what seemed natural; queuing up in line at a gate for a departing flight – even though it wasn't his. Most likely, Stan joined a group boarding the plane and just fit in. Thanks to security and the airlines, Stan was located quickly in Maui and kept safe until Paula could join him. Together, they boarded another plane for their final destination in Kauai. When Paula returned home, she realized that Stan needed to see a doctor for a diagnosis, and she needed to learn more about this condition.

TIP #7: Seek out a quiet place to wait for your flight

Again, if you have a long wait at the airport, consider purchasing a day pass to the airline's club or premium lounge. Buy the pass ahead of time, if you are able.

Take a look at the airport website prior to your trip. Identify places that may be quiet, perhaps a small museum or chapel. Find a smaller restaurant with fewer people. If tables are available toward the back of the restaurant, request to be seated away from the commotion of others passing by.

TIP #8: At the gate

As we've discussed, identify yourself to the gate agent and confirm that you will need early boarding or other accommodation, especially if you didn't confirm those requests at check-in.

Be sure to carry the companion card and don't be afraid to discreetly pass it to those around you as you wait, particularly if you see your person becoming anxious or upset.

TIP #9: Use early boarding

Even though you and your person may not have limitations in walking, you will benefit from early boarding and the added time to find your seats and settle in. Don't worry what others think when they see an able-bodied person joining a group of disabled adults to pre-board. Your goal is to stay close to your person and help them feel safe and secure.

TIP #10: Get comfortable once you board

Ideally, your person is seated by the window with you or your companion in the center seat. Now is the time for you to take a breath after braving a very busy airport! Have snacks and diversion activities readily available and ready to go. The boarding process may seem eternally long, even before taxiing out to the runway for takeoff.

CHAPTER 20

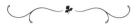

10 Tips for In-Flight/Connecting Flight, and Arrival

You are boarded and on your way. You may want to lead yourself and your loved one through a series of three to five long breath cycles (a slow breath in, followed by a long, slow exhale). The first one-third of the trip is now behind you. However, with packed planes and unexpected delays, you need to prepare for the next third – inflight, followed by connections and then arrival at your destination.

TIP #1: Encourage a brief rest or quieting activity

The airport has been very stimulating, but you're safely onboard and seated. Now is the time for a rest or quieting activity for 30 minutes to one hour (or more).

Noise-canceling headsets and/or the use of music can help calm your person. Put the window shade down once you are airborne and, since airplanes are often chilly, offer your person a light jacket or blanket.

TIP #2: Use what you learned in Chapter 9, *10 Tips for Keeping Your Person Occupied during Travel*

Alternating conversation with music, TV shows, movies, and favorite snacks will help the time pass.

TIP #3: Expect to hear repeated questions

Your loved one is likely to forget the destination or how long it will take to arrive. Don't get frustrated by these repeated questions. Try to answer patiently, as if you are hearing the question for the first time. Or, you can write the answer(s) to expected questions on a notecard and place it in a purse or a pocket. Let them know they have these 'reminders' on their notecard.

TIP #4: Prompt your person to use the toilet a few hours into the flight

Let the flight attendant know you may need to squeeze into the lavatory to assist, or that you will need to stand near the toilet to close the door or check in on your person. If you have a connecting flight and the time is tight, be sure to prompt toileting prior to landing.

TIP #5: Avoid alcohol during the flight as it may add to confusion

You may want to let the flight attendant know ahead of time that you are trying to avoid alcohol consumption for your person. With discretion, place the beverage order for your loved one. Think about ordering a 'mocktail,' for example, bloody Mary mix or club soda with a twist of lime or lemon.

TIP #6: Use your companion card

Remember the Companion Card you learned about in Chapter 1? While you're in-flight may be the perfect time to use it, especially if you need to discreetly inform other passengers of your person's behavioral expressions. Remember, this is also why it is important for the flight crew to know about your person, so they don't respond in a negative, unwanted manner.

TIP #7: Verify that a wheelchair and/or skycap has been requested at the arrival or connecting gate

Check with the gate agent at departure and again with the flight attendant during the flight.

TIP #8: Consider flight delays and close connections

Proactively speak to the gate agent and/or the flight attendants about how they can assist when there are unexpected delays. When booking flights, be sure that you have up to two hours between connecting flights to build in extra time for delays, toileting, etc.

It's important because it will minimize your stress. Remember, if you are stressed, your loved one will mimic your stress and add their own. Maybe this is time to take several deep breaths again.

TIP #9: Get assistance with your baggage

Your attention needs to stay on your person. There is growing fatigue in both of you. Your loved one will feel better if you are less weighed down by luggage and added stress. Pay for a skycap or ask a family member or friend to greet you in baggage claim to assist you with luggage.

TIP #10: Tuck in when you get to your destination

Expect more confusion this evening and even into the next day or two and factor it into your plans. For example, if you are cruising, attending a wedding or family reunion, you may want to arrive two days in advance to acclimate to a new time zone and location while incorporating your person's routine into the new location. Be sure you rest up, as well. This travel experience is a marathon, not a sprint. (*We'll go over this in more detail in Chapter 22, 10 Tips for Arriving at Your Destination.*)

CHAPTER 21

10 Tips for Cruising

Cruising is by far one of the favorite ways for people of all ages to travel. With so many choices, it can be overwhelming for first-time cruisers to know how to identify the best ship to meet their needs, whether traveling solo, with family, friends or in a group. An important benefit of cruising, for the person living with dementia and family, is that this full-service travel provides everything that might be needed, all under one roof. However, like other forms of travel, you will need to do some careful planning.

TIP #1: Shop for a cruise according to length and services available

Just as you have identified your goals for this trip (*please see Chapter 6, 10 Tips to Successful Travel Planning*), it is important to understand what type of cruise and ship will best suit your needs. With so many choices, it will be helpful to work with a travel agent who specializes in cruising and is knowledgeable about a wide range of options, including special needs.

In recent years, European river cruising has grown in popularity. However, it could be that getting to Europe to begin your trip will be too much for you and your loved one. Be realistic! You may need to stay stateside, but you can still have a great trip. There is a growing number of options for river cruises in the United States.

Likewise, with the growth of multi-generational cruising, it is essential to know which options will engage the kids while keeping the grandparent with dementia from becoming overwhelmed by too much noise, commotion or crowds. ***In other words, be careful and do your homework.***

While all ships may have accessible rooms, the focus is largely accommodating physical disability, ***not*** cognitive disability. While those physical disability services may be helpful, you will need to further explore exactly what they will mean for your person.

Like the airlines, there is no cruise industry standard for cognitive impairment. While children's programs (and specialty programs for autism) are common on many of the larger ships to give parents a break, there are no similar services for people living with dementia.

The web pages of some cruise lines will have an accessibility link that will take you to more information. When this is not readily available, ask your travel agent to get more information, or you can call the cruise line directly to learn more. A few cruise lines will request additional information from potential customers and will require a Special Needs Form to be completed at least thirty to sixty days prior to departure. Some cruise lines may also ask you for a medical provider's note to clear the person for travel.

As with airlines, be sure to communicate your person's needs so that the ship is prepared to receive them. When you check-in, use boarding assistance, confirm that any special needs are on file in your ship's records.

TIP #2: Smaller ships can be helpful to avoid lines and crowds

Many smaller ships (100 – 900 passengers) are considered premium or luxury brands and often come with added butler service and even added accommodations for medical equipment and services. Many will have an older group of passengers which may limit excess noise in common spaces including restaurants, bars, and pools.

Even when the ship is smaller, it will be helpful to know what types of disability services are available.

TIP #3: Work with your travel/cruise agent to book a room that meets your needs

As you select your cabin on the ship, you can use the same guidelines presented in Chapter 12, *10 Tips for Hotel Stays*. Ideally, you want your room to be laid out in a way that is similar to home and is located away from added noise or commotion.

For those with mobility issues, consider booking a disability-accessible room that may aid with bathing and other mobility needs. Travel agents and cruise ships can also proactively arrange for needs that range from hospital beds, to shower chairs, to portable oxygen and more. The added benefit: these aids can be delivered directly to the ship. Ships have a limited number of accessible rooms, so it is important to secure this type of accommodation well in advance of your trip.

When you book, look for a cabin located closer to the elevator to minimize walking, making it easier for your person to get around the ship.

TIP #4: Think through the dining experience

Cruising has the added benefit of multiple dining options. Yet, keep in mind that, by the moderate stage of dementia, most individuals will have a difficult time ordering from a menu. In this situation and with your help, the wait staff might make suggestions or even show your person a couple of featured dishes to make it easier to make a selection.

Buffets often work beautifully for the same reason. While your person may not remember the items on the menu, seeing the options in a buffet will allow them to select and eat what they enjoy. (Since buffets can be busy, try to visit before peak hours.) Let your wait staff know how they can best support your person's dining experience.

Sticking to your loved one's normal eating hours and their regular, home routine will be an immense help while cruising. If you are traveling with a group, let them know that the early dinner seating will be best; or, find a ship that provides flexible dining hours to accommodate the various needs and wants of the group.

Keep in mind the size of the dining table and the number of companions. A table with more than four to six others will become overwhelming to your person, as they struggle to keep pace with the conversation. Being seated in a quieter location, in a smaller table or near a window will make for a less distracting experience.

Make your dining requests in advance of your trip or on the very first day at sea. Help your dining partners to include your loved one in the conversation during dinner. One of the joys of eating with others is the socialization – something often lacking for those living with dementia.

Don't forget about room service. If you find your loved one is having an off-day or is more confused or fatigued, this is a perfect service, giving you both the chance to enjoy a meal in the quiet of your room.

TIP #5: Watch alcohol intake

While your person may have once enjoyed an evening cocktail, it will be important to limit the amount to the equivalent of one, six-ounce glass of wine; one, 12-ounce beer; or one-ounce of hard liquor. Find out if non-alcoholic beer or wine options are available. If not, some cruise lines will allow you to bring two bottles of wine per stateroom (of course, in this case, you'll be bringing non-alcoholic wine). This is another important thing to check *prior* to departure.

Since the bar and dining services are such a big part of the cruise experience, let your wait staff, sommelier or bartender know about your person's needs. With the variety of virgin cocktails available, the person can still enjoy a 'mocktail' in a glass that feels familiar and dignified while avoiding the added confusion that alcohol can bring.

TIP #6: Look for small or private excursions that avoid crowds and take less time

Some cruise lines are beginning to offer accessible excursions, but they are typically designed for those who use wheelchairs or scooters. Most of these outings are four or more hours, which can be too long for those with dementia. Scheduling a private excursion will be ideal.

A travel agent can be most helpful in finding private vendors who can support you and your person's needs. If scheduling a private tour with a group of family or friends, try to keep the group size under 10 people.

The best time for an excursion is mid-day – that way, you'll avoid lines when embarking and debarking the ship. In general, those with mild dementia can often tolerate up to four hours on an excursion, while those with moderate dementia will do best with excursions under two hours.

TIP #7: Once again, consider taking a travel companion

Throughout this book, we have discussed the importance of a travel companion, especially on extended trips. If you are the primary family caregiver, it is important for you to have some down time to relax and recoup from the daily demands. But without an identified companion, this will not happen, particularly if you are unable to safely leave your person unattended for a period of time.

Review Chapter 14, *10 Tips for Hiring a Travel Companion*, and use that advice to identify what you (and your loved one) may need in a cruise companion. Or consider booking a Dementia-Friendly Cruise that provides daily respite options for you and engagement for your loved one (more information is available at the end of this book under *Resources*).

TIP #8: Try to keep your usual routine intact while at sea

You know by now that routine creates comfort when time concepts are lost. While cruising, since everything around your person has changed, use your at-home routine to help them feel comfortable. This means:

- Eat your meals around the same time each day (or at the time you ordinarily would at home).

- Keep bedtime at about the same each night, or plan to encourage a late afternoon nap if you intend to enjoy late-night entertainment on the ship.

Remind anyone traveling with you that you are not being rigid – rather you are providing greater predictability for your loved one.

TIP #9: Think safety onboard and in ports

There is certainly a sense of greater safety when passengers are on board a ship. Yet, it is not the responsibility of the ship's staff to keep a watchful eye out for your loved one. While you may want to inform the staff of your person's dementia and seek out any additional ideas for safety, it is essential to plan ahead for any added safety needs.

With Wi-Fi readily available on most ships, combined with the growth and availability of GPS technology, some cruise lines are offering wearable technology that makes it easy for passengers to open the cabin door, make seamless payments and assist in finding their way around the ship.

Some cruise lines offer wearable technology for kids, so parents know where they are at any time. This same kind of service may be helpful for those with dementia, providing a safety net should you be separated from your person while onboard the ship. Inquire ahead of time to see if this is an option that might work for you and your person.

Some cruise lines also offer this sort of GPS technology for use while exploring the area during a land excursion while in port. As with any technology, make sure you know how to use it **before** venturing out.

Some families may elect to use GPS locator technology on their smartphones as a safety mechanism during cruising. If so, **make sure your loved one's phone is fully charged each day, that it is turned on, and is with them at all times**. Remember, phones only work if you have cell service available. Check with your cellphone carrier before the trip.

Another simple safety measure: make sure your person is wearing a neck lanyard with the cruise card or picture ID and cabin number. A wife who loved cruising with her husband took a picture of him each day with her cell phone so that, should they become separated, she could give an accurate description of him, including how he was dressed for the day.

As mentioned previously, bring along night lights to aid in finding the bathroom and, if you are concerned that your loved one will get up during the night and try to exit the room, consider bringing a door alarm. (*Please see Resources: Safety – Portable Door Locks.*)

TIP #10: Let the cruise staff know how they can help you and your person

The cruise industry is steeped in hospitality training intended to create a positive and comfortable experience for all. Yet, like the other forms of travel we've discussed, many cruise staffers have had little to no training about dementia. Thus, their ability to anticipate your needs will vary.

If you have not traveled with your person and are unsure how they will fare at sea, work with your travel agent or directly with the cruise line to determine which accessibility features will benefit you. Consider how to ease check-in and embarking/debarking; how to select dining preferences; and how to access additional safety features on the ship. Talk to your cabin steward, maître d' and other attendants directly, to ensure your person's needs are met.

CHAPTER 22

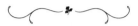

10 Tips for a Road Trip

Road trips are a favorite of many, offering more flexible travel for visiting family and friends and the chance to leisurely explore new places. In fact, about half of all road trips are taken each year to see family and friends, especially during holidays (https://newsroom.aaa.com/2019/03/100-million-americans-will-embark-on-family-vacations/).

Yet, the demands of long days on the road, coupled with frequent changes in location, can add to your person's confusion. While some family caregivers report success in this type of travel, others will need to carefully assess and plan for a road trip.

Consider the following tips:

TIP #1: Be realistic

Ask yourself if your loved one can truly handle a road trip. Just as you may have tried a staycation before embarking on a longer trip, you might want to see how your person will do on the road by first trying a day-long outing in your local area. Make sure your person is well-rested and start your travel at their best time of day.

Think carefully about your loved one's desire to help with driving. While in the early stage of dementia, many people are indeed able to drive in familiar locations, the added stress of unfamiliar roads may add to confusion and create safety concerns. Have your person assessed by a health professional first. If the professional indicates it is not a good idea for your person to drive, and yet they continue to insist on doing so, taking to the road may **not** be your best option.

TIP # 2: Plan each day carefully

Get out your map (or pull one up online) and plan ahead. Think about:

- Where you and your person can stop to use the restroom

- Where you can get a snack, beverage or meal, and

- Where you will spend the night.

Include a backup Plan B should you need to stop earlier due to fatigue, growing confusion and/or frustration (yours or your loved one). While you always want to book hotel rooms in advance, know whether you can cancel without penalty by calling the reservation center or speaking with the hotel directly.

TIP #3: Determine if a companion should join you

Road trips are demanding for the driver as you attend to the road and navigate traffic. Perhaps you need someone to help you with the driving or who can keep your person occupied. Be realistic as you think through your and your person's needs.

It's important to remember that, even if you once frequently traveled the road together, things are different now and **this trip will be different than road trips in the past.** To ensure you both enjoy this time together, by all means, consider hiring a companion to assist.

TIP #4: Let others know about your plans

It is important to let family and/or friends know of your plans and itinerary. You may also want to arrange for nightly check-ins to let someone know where you are in your journey. Using smart technology on your phone, you can even share your location as you go. It's a less intrusive way for people who care about you to keep track of your whereabouts and assist if there's an emergency.

TIP #5: Think safety: the car, your person, and you

Before you begin a road trip, be sure your car is in good repair. Have a mechanic check tire pressure, brakes, battery, hoses, and fluids.

Review your car insurance policy for roadside assistance, should you need it. In addition, think about carrying an emergency kit in your car. Your kit should include a flashlight with extra batteries, a tire gauge, tire iron, emergency flares or a reflector, a basic tool kit, gloves, and paper towels. You may also want to carry a basic first aid kit and extra drinking water. (For more car travel tips, please visit AAA at www.aaa.com and check the Resources section at the end of this book.)

It almost goes without saying that you will need a cell phone as you travel. These days, there is no reason to travel without one. Be sure to bring a charger and keep the phone charged throughout the trip. In your phone's settings, double-check to be sure your GPS is turned on for additional navigation support (in other words, don't expect your person to help you locate exits and addresses). If your loved one also has a phone, ensure it, too, is fully charged.

With constant changes in location during road trips, keep a watchful eye out for your loved one at all times. You may want to carry an 'occupied' sign to put on a restroom door if you need to go in to assist your person. As with other public restrooms, don't expect a stranger to watch your loved one while you use the restroom; your person is likely to ignore the guardian and walk away.

Be careful not to leave your loved one alone in the car. For some, that might mean not even for a brief moment. Take the keys with you, so your loved one does not spontaneously decide they want to drive.

If you are concerned that your person might open the door while the vehicle is moving, be sure to utilize the childproof locks. It may also be an indication that a companion should be present for added safety.

Whenever you find yourself worrying that your person might wander away during a trip, consider all the options available to assist with safety. Basic tips include:

- Ensure an identification card is located in a pocket, wallet, handbag or on a lanyard around your person's neck.

- Write your person's name and phone number on a shirt label.

- Enroll in the Alzheimer's Association Medic Alert + Safe Return program. For a small fee, it provides an identification bracelet or necklace, a personalized emergency wallet card and a 24-hour nationwide response system to aid law enforcement agencies in finding your person and reuniting them with you. An identification bracelet/necklace is also available for the caregiver.

- Research the wide range of trackable devices for added safety and subscribe well in advance of your trip. (*Please see Resources: Safety Products - GPS Technology for Wandering.*)

Since you have given careful thought and created a Plan B, make sure to use it if your person becomes increasingly confused, upset or belligerent – they may have reached their limit for the day. Ignoring these cues may create a safety issue. Instead, call it a day and focus on comfort strategies.

Never forget about yourself. You must also be in good condition to make a road trip. Be realistic about whether you are prepared to manage all of the driving, decisions, and engagement of your person along the way. If you are short-tempered and not prepared to hear repeated questions, look instead for a quicker mode of transportation or bring a companion. While road trips might have been fun in the past, they may now be too stressful for one or both of you.

TIP #6: Set reasonable limits for daily driving

Limit driving to no more than six hours each day. You will also want to plan to stop about every two hours to prompt use of the restroom, stretch, and/or get something to eat or drink.

If your loved one has been sleeping throughout most of the drive, don't be tempted to go further. It will be even more important to get to the planned destination for the day and keep your person awake for several hours before bedtime to minimize waking too early morning or in the middle of the night. You may determine along the way that your person can only tolerate four hours of driving at a time. If so, readjust your timeline and planned stops.

TIP #7: Bring along diversional activities

With the lost sense of time, even six hours of daily travel may seem eternally long for one or both of you. Plan ahead for diversional activities that are easy to manage and that you both enjoy.

Think about simple activities you've used in the past with the kids: keeping a list of state license plates, playing road trip travel Bingo using pictures rather than words, or enjoying an easy scavenger hunt in which you're looking for one item at a time. Before you leave, use your favorite online search engine to look for "road trip games" to find new ideas.

Remember, always keep these activities at a level intended for adults. Your loved one is not a child and will not engage if treated like one.

Audiobooks are another option. Consider short stories rather than those with long or challenging plots, since your person may have difficulty keeping pace with the storyline and characters. 'TED' and 'TEDx' Talks are generally shorter and offer interesting speakers covering a variety of topics. You can download them prior to your trip, knowing they may provide a pleasant diversion.

Finally, refer back to Chapter 9, *10 Tips for Keeping Your Person Occupied During Travel*. Remember that you can often use many of these same activities throughout the day and the duration of your trip.

TIP #8: Bring along extra supplies

One of the pleasures of road trips is indulging in treats along the way. Plan to bring plenty of favorite foods (even if they are unhealthy pleasures!) and beverages. Don't try to limit fluids during these multiple-day trips, since dehydration can lead to numerous and unwanted issues including urinary tract infections and constipation. While water is best, if your loved one does not enjoy water, then encourage fruit juices, sports drinks, or other non-caffeinated beverages. Use a travel cup with a straw and encourage your loved one to take a few sips every 30-minutes or so.

Bring along a supply of wet wipes for unexpected spills or washing hands. In addition, if your loved one uses an incontinence product or may be prone to an accident during travel, be sure to have extra products available, along with a readily accessible change of clothing in the car.

TIP #9: When you get to your destination, stay in a single location

Whether you are visiting family and friends or an intended vacation spot, find a single location for the duration of the trip, right up until you get back in the car to head home. Moving between hosts' homes or changing hotels to accommodate visiting family will add to your person's confusion. Be strategic and realistic, especially with family and friends who want you to stay with them. Help them to understand, in advance, what you need to make this a successful trip for your loved one. (*You may also want to review Chapter 6, 10 Tips for Successful Travel Planning.*)

TIP #10: Try to factor your person's routine into the day

It's true with just about any kind of travel – sticking to your general routine will help to keep you both grounded during the day. Well before the trip begins, think about how you will do this and communicate to others how they can implement your daily routine.

A Tale of Two Road Trips: One Successful – One Not!
The First Tale: Always at Home

Bud and his wife Mary Lou had grand plans for their retirement that included lots of travel. However, after Mary Lou was diagnosed with dementia, Bud knew that their plans needed to be adapted. Since the couple had four adult children and many grandchildren living across the U.S., they purchased an RV to provide the familiarity and predictability Bud knew would be essential for Mary Lou.

Bud carefully plans his travel around the kids and grandkids each year, while also wintering in a warmer location where they have come to make friends since Mary Lou's diagnosis.

Regardless of where they go, Bud follows the same routine with Mary Lou during the day. And, each night they return to the comfort of the RV, where Mary Lou feels safe and secure. Bud acknowledges that at some point this won't work, but for now, this form of travel has provided them both with what they need to make the most of enjoying family and friends.

The Second Tale: Way too Much

Frank and Lillian had loved to take road trips together over the years. Even though Lillian had moderate- stage dementia, Frank appreciated her gentleness and ability to go with the flow in groups.

When the couple was encouraged by their adult children to make a trip to visit the family back in Wisconsin, Frank decided this would be a great opportunity for the two of them. He carefully planned their days on the road, considering when and where they would stop to use the restrooms and get lunch. He also planned to limit daily travel time to six hours, checking into a hotel at the end of each day.

The couple enjoyed listening to favorite music and Frank gently reminded Lillian that they would be visiting their family in Wisconsin as she repeatedly questioned where they were going over the four-day trip.

This couple was so beloved by their three adult children, numerous siblings, and cousins that they graciously accepted more than a dozen invitations over their two-week stay. These invitations also included lodging in four different family homes. Frank noted growing confusion and irritability in Lillian but didn't want to cut the trip short.

Finally, the couple began to make their way home. But instead of the comfortable trip they enjoyed on the way to Wisconsin, Lillian became very agitated, often wanting to get out of the car. Frank found it more difficult to keep her occupied and distracted. She slept poorly in yet another four unfamiliar hotel locations on the way home – and so did he. Upon arriving home, an exhausted Frank could quickly see that the days of road trips had become a thing of the past.

CHAPTER 23

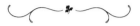

10 Tips When Arriving at Your Destination

Once you and your person have arrived at the intended destination, it is time to settle in for the rest of the day. Typically, when greeted by family and friends, we deposit our belongings in a room and start to catch up over a meal, often inviting other guests. While this sounds fantastic, it will only add to the growing fatigue and subsequent confusion in your person – creating problems you will see *that evening and up to three days later.*

On long trips that involve time zone changes, allow your person to acclimate to the new time zone. As you settle in to this new, temporary schedule, please apply what you've learned so far: pace yourself and use your person's usual daily routine to plan any outings and guide your commitments for each travel day.

These additional tips will also be helpful:

TIP #1: Inform family or friends ahead of time of the need for rest upon arrival and for the upcoming few days

This is critically important, especially for longer-duration travel such as lengthy flights or road trips. Fatigue will be present but perhaps masked by the excitement of seeing loved ones or arriving at a new destination. It's smart to resist the desire to join in for a family gathering. Instead, proceed at a slower pace, so your loved one gets the rest they need.

When taking a cruise or tour, arriving a couple of days in advance will give you and your person time to adjust to the time zone and be well-rested for your trip. Don't be in a rush to begin exploring. Ease into the new location and adhere to your person's regular routine as much as possible.

TIP #2: After pickup, go directly to your hotel or friend/family's home

Ask a family member to meet you at the airport and assist you to check into your hotel or settle in at their home. If friends or family aren't available, and rather than hailing a cab, arrange in advance for a hired driver to take you to your destination and assist with baggage as you check in. If you need to make a quick stop for beverages or snacks, do so on the way.

TIP #3: If staying with a family member or friend, ask them to get your person something to eat and drink, then allow them to rest while you settle in

When you arrive at a family's or friend's home, you can also use the first few minutes to provide information you might want to share with them to assist with your stay. While your person visits with family or friends upon arrival, you can use that time to unpack and settle in. But if fatigue is present, leave the bags until the next day. Just get out what you need for the evening.

TIP #4: Resist the temptation to get together with a group of family or friends for dinner

Of course, you've had a conversation with family members well in advance of your trip, so they know you need a quiet evening upon arrival. Whether dining in or out, the gathering should be small (ideally less than four people) and quiet.

If you're staying at a hotel, be sure you've booked a room at a place with a small restaurant or, better yet, where room service is available. Plan ahead, should you need to order out. Remember, you're tired, too! The easier it is to settle in and get a nice meal, the better.

TIP #5: If you do go to dinner, ask family or friends to excuse themselves for the evening

While it may be way too early for family/friends to go to bed, adjourning early will allow you and your person to go to your room – whether it's at a private home or a hotel – and settle in for the evening. Remember, you might need to prompt your loved one to "call it a day."

TIP #6: Begin your nighttime routine as if at home

As I've said many times before, try to use the same routines in your new location that you use at home. Routines are comfortable and familiar. And with your person's lost sense of time, this will provide them with the space and time needed to wind down and get ready for bed.

TIP #7: If your person insists on staying up longer, have them listen to music, leaf through a newspaper or magazine or watch non-violent/non-news shows

Most likely, you've got your bag of tricks and diversions close at hand (please review Chapter 9, *10 Tips for Keeping Your Person Occupied during Travel*). Try to engage your loved one in an activity that is not too stimulating. Avoid the temptation to turn the TV to the local news station; the emphasis on bad news can create unwanted stimulation and agitation.

TIP #8: Place night lights in the bathroom and bedroom

Bring along a few night lights, since the room in which you and your loved one are staying in will be unfamiliar. If you are staying in a home without an attached bathroom, be sure to light the hallway, too. If a stairway is nearby, you'll need extra vigilance to avoid a fall.

Remember to let your person sleep on the same side of the bed as they do at home. Place familiar objects at the bedside to enhance that sense of home.

TIP #9: Cue your person to use the toilet before bedtime

Since the environment is new, the usual 'cues' to take care of business may be lost. You might try saying something like, "Let's check out the bathroom to see if we have everything we need." Or, "Let's go to the bathroom before we go to bed!" Either way, ensure your person has the opportunity to see and use the toilet before bedtime.

TIP #10: Be prepared for some added confusion while your person settles into the new location

Sticking to your familiar home routine for meals, getting ready for the day, TV shows, daily walks, etc., will help to ease your person into this new environment. This also means you may need to limit the number of visits with family and friends or spread them over a longer period of time.

During the first couple of days on a trip, you may also want to limit the number of tours or excursions you join. Use your best judgment and let the person's "behavioral expressions" be your guide to know if they are fatigued or overwhelmed. When fatigue and overwhelm strike, just back off a bit and take things more slowly.

CHAPTER 24

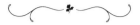

10 Tips for Your Return Home (or When Your Guests Leave)

It is not uncommon to find that the person with dementia does exceptionally well during travel or during visits with family and friends. In fact, many caregivers will report that the person seemed "almost normal." When this happens, it's a great indicator of your person's ability to draw upon long-held social skills and can be a reason for celebration.

However, upon your return home or after the visitors leave, your person can suddenly develop increased confusion. This will, no doubt, take you by surprise. Even when there's no discernible change, it is still essential to ease back into your normal routine. **_Be aware_**: this return to normalcy can take several days, even up to a week or more.

A Treasured Homecoming

Hanna had been living with Alzheimer's disease for about three years when her family from Finland called to announce they would soon host a party celebrating Hanna's father's 95th birthday. Hanna began talking with her husband, Don, about making one last trip home to see her dad. After a great deal of thought, and seeking guidance from Hanna's neurologist and nurse, Don set out to plan and execute a demanding trip that would last more than two weeks.

Don proceeded to do everything right. He booked business class tickets for the couple since he had been advised that this additional space would support Hanna's ability to sleep during the long flight. Anticipating a layover of several hours in New York, Don purchased a day pass to the airline's club, offering an escape from the noisy airport and a quieter place for the two of them to wait.

As part of his planning, Don had informed Hanna's family about her condition. He let them know that she was frequently confused and a bit less talkative than what they'd remembered. He shared that nighttime was particularly difficult for Hanna and that she needed quiet space, along with short rest periods throughout the day.

Since Hanna's sister insisted the couple stay in her home, Don was clear in his pre-travel communication. He shared that, once they arrived, he and Hanna would appreciate a quiet dinner with the family and would then excuse themselves to unpack and settle in for the night. He asked the family to be flexible and note when Hanna became overwhelmed, and to aid him by assisting her to a quiet space or ending the activity.

Thanks to Don, everyone was prepared to play a role in her care and the whole family enjoyed a splendid visit.

Their return trip to the U.S. proved to be a bit more challenging. Throughout the flight home, Hanna kept asking Don, "Where are we?" And despite his attempts to gently explain the situation, this repetition continued throughout most of the flight.

The return flight required a layover in Atlanta, but in this case, the airline did not have a club. In a smart move, Don sought out the airport chapel which provided a quiet place for them to rest until the next leg of their trip home.

Once home, Hanna was quite confused. Don had been advised that this could happen and that the best medicine would be to limit stimulating activities and get Hanna back into their familiar routine. Although it took two weeks, Hanna returned to her usual functioning.

During a routine visit to Hanna's Memory Clinic, the pair was elated to report to her doctor and nurse that they'd enjoyed a fabulous trip and a wonderful family visit. They reminisced about the familiar sights and favorite foods they'd savored. Hanna was so appreciative of her husband's efforts to take this treasured final trip to her homeland. And Don was pleased he'd followed the sage travel advice he'd been given.

TIP #1: Come home to the essentials

If possible, ask family or friends to stop by the grocery store and pick up some familiar food items before your return home. This doesn't mean you need to be fully stocked but having items for breakfast and lunch the next day will minimize your stress and ease your return.

TIP #2: Go directly home and rest

If family or friends are picking you up from the airport, have them take you directly home. Resist the urge to invite them in or to stay and hear about your trip.

And if family guests were staying with you in your home, recognize that it may be too much for you to drive them to the airport. If you do, plan to drop them at the departure area and head back home.

TIP #3: Get back into your routine immediately!

Whether you're returning home, or your houseguests are leaving, and no matter what time of day, ***re-start your familiar, comforting routine immediately!*** This will be very important in assisting your loved one to adjust and reset their internal time clock.

TIP #4: Allow for added rest and/or naps

Even if your return falls early in the day, having added rest and a slower, quieter day will be good for both of you. Resist the need to start laundry, go through the mail, or do any of innumerable chores that beckon you. It can all wait a bit longer!

Encourage a nap in the afternoon. It may help with evening confusion (often referred to as ***sundowning***) and may help to keep your person awake later into the evening.

TIP #5: Invite your person to assist you, if possible

Minor tasks such as taking the garbage out, washing a few dishes or sweeping the floor give a sense of purpose to your person and may also provide you an opportunity to get a few things done without your person hovering.

TIP #6: Eat in or order out

Keeping it simple will be best for both of you. Whether you eat a sandwich, heat up a frozen dinner or have a pizza delivered, a quiet meal at home supports your person as they move back to the comfort of the routine.

TIP #7: Use evening rituals

Your loved one will be tired and may want to go to bed early. Yet, you'll both do better if you try to keep your person awake until at least 8:00 p.m. To do it, use evening routines such as watching a favorite TV show, leafing through a magazine, listening to music or assisting with a chore. This way, you can avoid seeing your person wide awake at 3:00 or 4:00 a.m., ready to start their day.

TIP #8: Don't forget that you need your rest too

You've been doing double-duty, ensuring your travel went smoothly or keeping your houseguests entertained. Recognize that it's imperative for you to rest and recharge your own batteries. Allow yourself to go to bed when your person does and plan to take a nap whenever you get the chance.

TIP #9: Limit errands and appointments

Over the coming days, try keeping errands outside of the home to a minimum. You may need to decline social activities for a few days until your person is back into the familiar groove of home. Let the people around you know how they can support you – perhaps planned calls from friends and family can keep you connected as your person transitions from travel to home life.

TIP #10: Expect confusion

Accept that your person's confusion will pass and with your help, ***things will return to normal***. As they do, you can relive your special trip by sharing pictures, stories, and mementos with family and friends.

In time, you can evaluate your trip to figure out what worked, what could use some tweaking, and how you will plan for the next trip or visit in the future.

Two Days Later....
After her husband Dean's dementia diagnosis, Lisa became a regular attendee at her local Alzheimer's Association support group meeting. On one particular meeting day, Lisa reported to her group about the couple's recent visit to see their children in New Jersey.

Lisa was delighted that Dean was so engaged during the visit. While he was not able to remember the grandchildren's names, he got by using his social charms and the special nicknames he'd give to each of them. Lisa noted that her own adult children were delighted with their dad's ability and even questioned his dementia diagnosis. Aside from a bit of verbal repetition, they said, "He seems normal."

Yet, Lisa shared that on the second day after their return home, Dean was very confused and insisted on using the car for an errand, forgetting he hadn't driven in over a year. She was taken by surprise and had to hide the car keys until the confusion cleared several days later. It helped her to hear, from several others in the support group, that their affected family members often had a similar response to travel.

Several group members also mentioned that during family visits, their loved ones living with dementia would act normal. Yet, as soon as the visit came to an end and the family pulled away, their person's dementia would return, just as before. They sympathized with Lisa and encouraged her to get back into Dean's daily routine. They also suggested that, now that the trip was over, she had the perfect opportunity to think through what she might do differently in advance of the next trip, including asking for more support from her adult kids.

CHAPTER 25

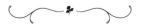

10 Tips for Creating Memories

Among the great benefits of travel is the opportunity to create new memories or revisit old ones. Just because your person is living with dementia and their memory is changing, don't allow this to diminish the possibility they may be able to form new memories to cherish, if even for a short time.

As we've seen, during travel it is not uncommon for the person's former and social self to shine through, allowing family and friends to see someone they have cherished. At the same time, it could be that the details of an old memory fade or a well-rehearsed story changes. If your loved one is happy telling a story, join them in enjoying that happiness. Through it all, remember that you, too, are also creating and adding to your own memory book. Take time to capture and cherish these special moments.

TIP #1: Live in the moment

While Alzheimer's disease and related dementias are considered "diseases of memory," they do not take away from your person's ability to enjoy the ***now.***

For some affected by this disease, the oldest memories drift away over time; for others, it's the ability to recall what happened a moment ago that disappears in a flash. This is why being fully present with the moments happening now, right in front of us, can be such a gift.

As you travel with your loved one, patiently learn to be present in each moment along the way. Try to relax and put aside what has not gone as planned or what you are worried about for tomorrow. This trip is precious as the two of you (and/or family and friends) enjoy the 'now' as it is and form new, precious memories that will sustain you through your remaining time together, and beyond.

TIP #2: Take pictures and videos along the way

You've heard the expression, "a picture is worth a thousand words." Smartphones have made it simple to capture the everyday moments that convey a memory, especially when words can't do it justice. So, whether you bring a camera, video recorder or just your phone, ***use it!***

And while pictures of beautiful places are wonderful, most of us are enthralled by looking at photos of those we love most. Take snapshots that include you, your person and others you care about. This is a part of the story you will tell now and in the future.

TIP #3: Document your journey

Don't forget to take a small notebook and pen on your trip, or to use your phone to take notes along the way. During your trip, spend a few moments each day jotting notes about the places you visited and the experiences you shared. Or, if others are traveling with you, ask them to record some observations from each day. Please don't wait until the end of the trip to try to recall all that you did – the days will begin to run together in your own memory.

Once home, you can combine notes and pictures to tell the story of your journey.

TIP #4: Buy souvenirs or pick up mementos during your trip

Most of us have a collection of seashells, an old baseball, a doll or postcards from family members. We keep these precious keepsakes because each tells a story – a potent and positive memory from the past.

You probably don't need any additional 'treasures' in your home, yet souvenirs or simple mementos serve as a wonderful reminder of a special time and place.

So, find a souvenir or memento that represents the trip. Use them as you revisit the trip with your person. Coupled with a few pictures and stories, these trinkets add to the joy of retelling the tales of your travel. And for some living with dementia, they will remember and connect to these special trinkets in ways you may not have anticipated.

TIP #5: Talk about the fun you've had

We all love to hear or tell a good story. Stories often represent shared experiences and can trigger the imagination. Your trip is no different.

Over the days and weeks after you've traveled, incorporate the story of your trip into your daily conversation. Give your person time to follow along and connect to the story. Ask them to join in and add to it – even if their version is very different than what actually happened. The joy is in telling and hearing the story.

If your person enjoys participating, continue to use this story for as long as possible. It's a beautiful way to revisit a fun destination or recall precious time spent with family and friends.

TIP #6: Create a photo book when you return

As we've discussed, photos, coupled with your stories and mementos, allow for greater connections for your person.

There are many software options available that make it easy to upload photos from your phone and design a unique photo book. Remember to use a lot of pictures of people you visited or met along the way. If it's important to you, you can label these individuals and write a simple story to go with each picture.

Since your work as a caregiver often leaves you pressed for time, consider asking your children or grandchildren to put together a photo book for you. If you're using standard film, have it developed and enlist the kids in making an old-fashioned scrapbook. Remember that, for your person, the chance to hold a book of photos may be far more powerful and engaging than just looking at them on a computer, phone or tablet.

TIP #7: Tell stories to others about your travels

You are sharing the memories for both of you, so don't be afraid to tell your stories to others. This will bring good memories back for you and will help family and friends learn more about the trip or visit you completed.

These stories can also provide a way for your family and friends to interact with your loved one. Encourage them to ask your person simple questions about the trip. Coupled with a picture, it might trigger a memory or fun response, allowing your loved one to join in on the storytelling.

There is a growing number of storytelling programs for people living with dementia that allow them to participate and build or add to a story. Consider locating a similar program near you. It could be a great way to give your person the opportunity to tell a story and bask in the great feelings associated with sharing it with a new audience.

TIP #8: Look at photos and mementos

Keep your photo book and mementos on a coffee or kitchen table – with luck, they will prompt your person to look. This also gives you a conversation starter and can serve as a pleasant activity – especially while you are preparing dinner or having some quiet time before bedtime.

TIP #9: Laugh about stories along the way

Laughter has been called the "best medicine" for a reason. It releases chemicals in our brains that help us feel better immediately. And when you laugh, your person is likely to laugh along with you.

Most of us love to recite funny stories from the past. You likely had some good laughs during your trip and can revisit them with your person and others. Rarely do trips or events go off without a few hiccoughs along the way, so laughing at the things that didn't go right will often help you feel better and bring delight to your person.

Whether it has to do with travel or not, take time to laugh each day – whether looking at pictures, telling a funny story, or watching something funny on TV. Laughter is good for both of you.

TIP #10: Celebrate your trip!

Whether this marks a trip that will encourage a few more in the future or defines a moment when this joint travel will end, the fact is: *you did it!* Give yourself credit for all the planning that went into it. Take note of what you learned and what you might do differently the next time. Either way, you made it!

A Final Adventure

Angie decided it was time for one last family trip with her dad, whose Alzheimer's disease was progressing. She planned a final trip to a beautiful National Park in their home state and included her mom, dad, and her sister who would serve as an additional travel companion.

Angie's dad had been an avid outdoorsman and her mom had always enjoyed joining in his adventures. Together, they experienced this beautiful park, took lots of pictures and reminisced about their favorite memories of family travel throughout their four-day trip.

When Angie returned home, she decided to memorialize the trip by creating a photo book of the adventure. When her dad could no longer remember the trip, she continued to use the book as a way to engage him whenever she visited.

Watching his precious reactions inspired her to design another photo album. Angie knew her dad was primarily recalling experiences from his younger years. Her goal was to transport him back to a time that was more familiar.

Fortunately, Angie's mom had squirreled away dozens of old photos. There were shots of her dad with his own parents and siblings, others from his time in the military, and still more from the early days of his career as a civil engineer. She added images of her mom and dad from their early years of marriage, along with photos of Angie and her siblings as young children. Since words no longer made sense, Angie was sure to select pictures that each told their own story.

Angie and her entire family began to use this photo book during every visit with their dad. Angie's mom found the book also helped him throughout his day, particularly when he began to get restless or upset. She would re-introduce the book to him by saying, "Look at these wonderful pictures!" She would invite him to join her on the couch and soon he began carefully looking at the pictures and slowly turning the pages. These 'time travels' remained important to all of them until the end of his life.

Conclusion

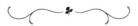

While the diagnosis of Alzheimer's disease or a related dementia will certainly be life changing, it is essential to stay focused on the possibilities that still remain in your loved one, now through the end of this life and your time together.

As I expressed at the beginning of this book, I firmly believe that it is possible to live well with dementia. And for many, traveling to new places and/or enjoying continued relationships with family and friends is more than just possible – it is good medicine for your person and for you.

I hope that, after reading this book in its entirety or just those sections that are most pertinent to your situation, you and your person will find the best possible options for living in the moment, enjoying each other's company and making new memories, whether through travel or by making the most of life wherever you are right now.

Our days and lives are made of single moments that create who we are and become our story. While memories may fade for your person, may they stay robust for you and others as you recount the joy of a life well-lived. Life is a journey and so is caring for a person living with dementia.

Please don't give up on the moments or the idea of creating new memories.

Moments matter.

May you find joy in your journey.

Traveling well with dementia is possible.

Resources

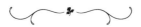

Alzheimer's Disease and Related Dementias

Alzheimer's Association (National): http://www.alz.org/
Provides access to a wealth of caregiver information and education, current research and enrollment to the ***Medic Alert + Safe Return*** program. This link can also help you find your local chapter.

- **24 Hour Helpline: (800) 272-3900**

Alzheimer's Disease Education and Referral Center (ADEAR):
http://www.nia.nih.gov/alzheimers

Provides current, comprehensive Alzheimer's disease information and resources from the National Institute on Aging for professionals and family caregivers.

- **ADEAR: (800) 438-4380** (Monday – Friday, 8:30 a.m. – 5:00 p.m. EST)

- **Email support:** adear@nia.nih.gov

Association for Frontotemporal Degeneration: http://www.theaftd.org/

Provides disease-specific information and help for those with Frontotemporal diseases.

- **Helpline: (866) 507-7222 (**Leave a message and someone will get back to you, generally within 24 hours on weekdays.)

- **Email support:** info@theaftd.org

Lewy Body Dementia Association, Inc.: http://www.lbda.org/

Provides disease-specific information for caregivers about Lewy Body Dementia.

Caregiver Link Helpline: (800) 539-9767

Email support: support@lbda.org

General Caregiver Services and Respite Care

Area Agencies on Aging: www.n4a.org

Provides information and referral for services for seniors by county across the United States. Includes information about home-delivered meals and caregiver respite sources. This link will connect you to your local Area Agency on Aging, many of which have local helplines.

Centers for Medicare and Medicaid Services (CMS): http://www.medicare.gov/nursinghomecompare

- **1-800-MEDICARE (1-800-633-4227)**

CMS offers a way to compare hospitals, nursing homes, and home care services on its website.

Please note: you can also connect to the agency in your state that is responsible for regulation and oversight of care facilities. You have the right to review at recent surveys (inspections) for nursing homes, assisted living communities, home health care agencies, and adult day health care.

The name of the agency will vary by state. For a list that includes agency names in all 50 states, please visit https://www.after55. com/blog/assisted-living-regulation-agencies-by-state/.

Eldercare Locator: www.eldercare.aci.gov
National program that is a public service of the U.S. Administration on Aging to help you locate a range of services in your area, including respite for caregivers.

- **(800) 677-1116** (Monday – Friday, 9am – 8pm EST)

- **Email Support:** eldercarelocator@n4a.org

National Academy of Elder Law Attorneys, Inc.: www.naela.org
Professional association of attorneys who are dedicated to improving the quality of legal services specific to older adults and people with special needs. This site can help you find an elder law attorney in your area. (Online only.)

National Adult Day Services Association: www.nadsa.org
Provides state-by-state help in finding local adult day care services. It also provides a list of questions to ask when visiting centers.

- **(877) 745-1440**

- **Email:**info@nadsa.org

National Respite Locator Service: www.respitelocator.org
Helps caregivers and professionals locate respite services in their communities. Includes an informative guide on how to choose respite care.

Dementia Specific Products for Activities, Clothing, Incontinence Care

Alzheimer's Store: http://www.alzstore.com/
Online store provides activity, caregiving, and safety products that are useful for people with all stages of dementia.

- **(800) 752-3238**

- **Email support:** contact@alzstore.com

Best Alzheimer's Products: http://www.best-alzheimers-products.com/
Online store that provides ideas and activity products for caregivers can use to engage with their loved ones.

- **(877) 300-3021**

- **(847) 223-3021**

- info@best-alzheimers-products.com

Buck and Buck: www.buckandbuck.com
Online store for adaptive and dignified clothing and footwear for people living with dementia or disabilities.

- **(800) 458-0600**

Comfort Plus: www.comfortplusonline.com
Online store specializing in incontinence products, bathroom and bedroom safety, and hygiene supplies. They provide free samples of their adult diapers, briefs, and other incontinence products, to ensure you are selecting the best product for your person.

- **(888) 656-8055**

MindCARE Store: www.mindcarestore.com

Online store that provides memory care and safety products for seniors.

- **(312) 543-3334**

- **Email support:** contact@MindCareStore.com

Safety Products

Portable Door Locks:

There are numerous, commercially available devices that can be used at home or during travel to alert you if your person is trying to leave the room without your knowledge. Most can be purchased online and range in price from $10 to $30. For travel, look for a product that is lightweight and can be easily placed on or off the door. Search for:

- Doberman Security Portable Door Alarm

- Lewis N Clark Travel Door Alarm

- Door Guard Alarm with Mini LED Light (Slips over doorknob and alarms if the door handle is moved.)

GPS Technology for Wandering:

There is a growing category of technology that provides life-saving tracking devices in the form of watches, pendants or necklaces, GPS tiles or shoe inserts. While there are numerous products available, consider each carefully to support the dignity and needs of your person.

Note: many of the devices will also have subscription fees and may not support international travel. Some require the person wearing the device to initiate the response by pushing a button and may best support those with mild dementia.

Wristwatch:

Adiant Mobile: www.adiantmobile.com

GPS locator watch connects to any smartphone.

- **(877) 980-4477**

- **Email support:** sales@adiantmobile.com

Medical Guardian: www.medicalguardian.com

Provides GPS tracking in the U.S. only, two-way text to speech messaging, and reminders for medications and appointments. Family members can download an app to track their person.

- **(800) 864-7173**

Necklace/Pendant:

Life Alert: www.lifealert.com/

Can be worn as a pendant or carried in a purse/pocket, this device has a 10-year battery and can detect falls and has a GPS device. **Note:** your person must push a button to activate the system, which is a limitation for those with moderate dementia.

- **(800) 360-0329**

Mindme: http://www.mindme.care/

This device can be worn as a pendant or carried in a pocket or purse. It uses GPS technology and does not require the person living with dementia to activate the system. It has a 48-hour battery life.

- **(914) 205-4234**

Shoe insert:

SmartSole: www.gpssmartsole.com

A GPS tracker is hidden in a shoe insole and provides online smartphone tracking through an app. It does not require the person to remember to carry or wear it daily. The device must be recharged daily.

- **(213) 489-3019**

Other wearable solutions:

AngelSense: www.angelsense.com

Portable GPS device that can be attached to a person's clothing, allowing the caregiver to track the person in both indoor and external locations. This device works throughout the U.S. and Canada.

- **(646) 770-2950**

PocketFinder: www.pocketfinder.com

Tracker device that can be carried on a keychain or in a purse and provides GPS technology allowing caregivers to use Google Maps on a smartphone to locate their family member.

- **(866) 726-7543**

Trax: www.traxfamily.com

Tracker device for a keychain or as a wrist strap sends the person's location to the caregiver's smartphone.

- support@traxfamily.com

Car Safety Products

There are numerous products that provide comprehensive options for road trips. They can be purchased online and in big box and auto stores.

Kolo Sports Premium Auto Emergency Kit

This compact kit contains 113 items you may need during a road trip in case of emergency and includes everything from battery cables, tire puncture repairs to roadside warning triangles. A first aid kit is also included.

- http://kolosports.com/instructions/automotive-roadside-assistance-first-aid-kit/

Lifeline AAA Excursion Road and First Aid Kit

This 76-piece kit includes products needed for a car or truck, along with a first aid kit.

- http://www.lifelinefirstaid.com/product/86

Thrive Roadside Assistance Emergency Kit

An all-weather kit with products that don't require batteries for use. Includes signage to signal for help, emergency vest and tow gear, along with a first aid kit.

- https://www.thrivebrandproducts.com/products/thrive-roadside-assistance-auto-emergency-kit-first-aid-kit-square-bag-contains-jumper-cables-tools-reflective-safety-triangle-and-more-ideal-winter-accessory-for-your-car-truck-camper

Dementia Friendly Cruising and Travel Resources

Elite Cruises and Vacations, LLC: www.elitecruisesandvacation-stravel.com

This travel company, owned and operated by a Registered Nurse (RN), focuses on creating travel opportunities for people living with dementia and other disabilities. Travel includes RN support and options for caregiver respite.

- **(888) 826-6836**

U.S. Department of Transportation: https://www.trans-portation.gov/individuals/aviation-consumer-protection/general-travel-tips-persons-disabilities

This site provides a variety of travel tips for people traveling with physical and mental disabilities. It provides access to a wide range of practical ideas and education materials.

References

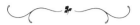

AAA. https://newsroom.aaa.com/2019/03/100-million-americans-will-embark-on-family-vacations

Alzheimer's Association. 2019 Alzheimer's Disease Facts and Figures. Alzheimer's Dementia 2019;15(3):321-87. Alzheimer's Association. 2019 Alzheimer's Disease Facts and Figures.

Global Coalition on Aging. (2018). Destination Healthy Aging: The Physical, Cognitive and Social Benefits of Travel. https://globalcoalitiononaging.com/wp-content/uploads/2018/07/destination-healthy-aging-white-paper_final-web.pdf. Accessed June 25, 2019.

Hall, G., & Buckwalter, K. (1987). Progressively lowered stress threshold: a conceptual model for care of adults with Alzheimer's disease. *Archives of Psychiatric Nursing, 1*(6), 399-406.

Hall, G. (2007). Travel Guide for People with Dementia. Produced by Banner Alzheimer's Institute.

Subramaniam, H. (2019). Co-morbidities in dementia: time to focus more on assessing and managing co-morbidities. Age and Ageing, 48(3), 314-315. https://doi.org/10.1093/ageing/afz007. Accessed June 25, 2019.

U.S. Travel Association. (2019). U.S. Travel Answer Sheet. https://www.ustravel.org/system/files/media_root/

document/Research_Fact-Sheet_US-Travel-Answer-Sheet.pdf. Accessed June 25, 2019.